# Colposcopy

## A Practical Guide

Second Edition

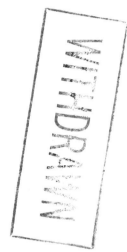

# Colposcopy

## A Practical Guide

### Second Edition

**Mahmood I. Shafi**
Consultant Gynaecological Surgeon and Oncologist, Addenbrooke's Hospital, Cambridge University Hospitals NHS Foundation Trust, Cambridge, UK

**Saloney Nazeer**
Consultant WHO Collaborating Centre in Education and Research in Human Reproduction, Geneva Foundation for Medical Education and Research, Geneva, Switzerland

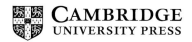

# CAMBRIDGE
## UNIVERSITY PRESS

University Printing House, Cambridge CB2 8BS, United Kingdom

Published in the United States of America by Cambridge University Press, New York

Cambridge University Press is part of the University of Cambridge.

It furthers the University's mission by disseminating knowledge in the pursuit of education, learning and research at the highest international levels of excellence.

www.cambridge.org
Information on this title: www.cambridge.org/9780110766782

First edition © Fivepin 2006
Second edition © M. I. Shafi and S. Nazeer 2012

First published by Fivepin, 2006
Second edition published by Cambridge University Press, 2012
Reprinted 2013

Printed in the United Kingdom by Bell and Bain Ltd

*A catalogue record for this publication is available from the British Library*

*Library of Congress Cataloguing in Publication data*
Shafi, Mahmood.
Colposcopy : a practical guide / Mahmood Shafi, Saloney Nazeer. – 2nd ed.
  p. ; cm.
Includes bibliographical references and index.
ISBN 978-1-107-66782-2 (pbk.)
I. Nazeer, Saloney.  II. Title.
[DNLM: 1. Colposcopy – methods.   2. Cervix Uteri – pathology.   3. Uterine Cervical Diseases – diagnosis.
4. Vagina – pathology.   5. Vaginal Diseases – diagnosis. WP 250]
618.1′407545–dc23

                                                                                    2011049750

ISBN 978-1-107-66782-2 Paperback

This book is dedicated to the love and support of our respective parents – Mohammed Shafi, Alam Begum Shafi; Mohammed Akhtar Khan and Nusrat Akhtar.

# Contents

# Glossary of terms

| | |
|---|---|
| AGC | Atypical glandular cells |
| AIS | Adenocarcinoma in situ |
| ALO | Actinomyces-like organisms |
| ASC-H | Atypical squamous cells, cannot exclude HSIL |
| ASC-US | Atypical squamous cells of undetermined significance |
| ATZ | Atypical transformation zone |
| BSCCP | British Society for Colposcopy and Cervical Pathology |
| BV | Bacterial vaginosis |
| CCI | Clinico–colposcopic index |
| CGIN | Cervical glandular intraepithelial neoplasia |
| CIN | Cervical intraepithelial neoplasia |
| CIS | Carcinoma in situ |
| CT | Computed tomographic scan |
| CTZ | Congenital transformation zone |
| $CO_2$ | Carbon dioxide |
| DNA | Deoxyribonucleic acid |
| DES | Diethylstilboestrol |
| ECC | Endocervical curettage |
| EFC | European Federation of Colposcopy |
| EMPD | Extramammary Paget's disease |
| FIGO | Federation Internationale de Gynecologie et d'Obstetrique |
| FNA | Fine-needle aspiration |
| 5FU | 5-Fluorouracil |
| HAART | Highly active antiretroviral therapy |
| HIV | Human immunodeficiency virus |
| HPV | Human papilloma virus |
| hrHPV | High-risk human papilloma virus |
| HSIL | High-grade squamous intraepithelial lesion |
| HSV | Herpes simplex virus |
| IFCPC | International Federation for Cervical Pathology and Colposcopy |
| ISSVD | International Society for the Study of Vulvovaginal Disease |
| IUCD | Intrauterine contraceptive device |
| IVU | Intravenous urogram |
| LBC | Liquid-based cytology |
| LCR | Ligase chain reaction |
| LEEP | Loop electrosurgical excision procedure |
| LLETZ | Large loop excision of the transformation zone |
| LS | Lichen sclerosus |
| LSIL | Low-grade squamous intraepithelial lesion |
| MRI | Magnetic resonance imaging |
| NETZ | Needle excision of transformation zone |
| NOS | Not otherwise specified |
| OR | Odds ratio |
| Pap smear | Papanicolaou smear |
| PCR | Polymerase chain reaction |
| PET | Positron emission tomography |
| PID | Pelvic inflammatory disease |
| QA | Quality assurance |
| SCC | Squamous cell carcinoma |
| SCJ | Squamocolumnar junction |
| SIL | Squamous intraepithelial lesion |
| STD | Sexually transmitted disease |
| SWETZ | Straight-wire excision of transformation zone |
| TBS | The Bethesda System |
| TNM | Tumor, node, metastasis |
| TZ | Transformation zone |
| VaIN | Vaginal intraepithelial neoplasia |
| VIN | Vulvar intraepithelial neoplasia |
| VLP | Virus-like particle |
| WHO | World Health Organization |

# Basic principles of colposcopy

Atypical cervical cytology or positive test for high-risk human papilloma virus (hrHPV), especially if it is persistent, may indicate the presence of abnormality on the cervix. Naked eye visualization will only detect invasive disease but cannot differentiate preinvasive disease from the normal cervix. In this situation colposcopic examination is important.

## Indications for colposcopy

Ideally all women with abnormal cervical cytology and/or positive hrHPV should undergo colposcopic assessment to identify those with and those without any clinically visible lesions. This allows clinical verification of the cervical cytology and hrHPV report. In those with an atypical lesion, the colposcope can aid diagnosis and management as appropriate. In those women where no atypical lesions are visualized, they can have a less stringent follow-up schedule often in the community setting.

Indications for colposcopy:

- Borderline (atypical squamous cells of undetermined significance, ASC-US) nuclear abnormalities on three occasions or single ASC-US with positive hrHPV test as triage.
- Mildly dyskaryotic cytology (low-grade squamous intraepithelial lesion, LSIL) with positive hrHPV test as triage if available. If HPV testing is not available, then referral after two consecutive mildly dyskaryotic cytology samples (LSIL) is acceptable practice.
- Moderate or severe dyskaryosis (high-grade squamous intraepithelial lesion, HSIL), with or without hrHPV status.
- Cytology suggestive of malignancy.
- Glandular abnormalities, irrespective of severity.
- Any degree of cytological abnormality or hrHPV positivity in women who have previously undergone treatment for cervical intraepithelial neoplasia (CIN).

- Repeated (three consecutive) unsatisfactory cervical cytology reports.
- Post-coital bleeding after age 40 if cancer suspected.
- Intermenstrual bleeding or persistent vaginal discharge if cancer suspected.
- Suspicious cervix suggestive of malignancy regardless of the cytology report. This may include an abnormal feeling cervix on bimanual examination.
- Lesions affecting the cervix e.g. condyloma acuminata which may have associated preinvasive or invasive disease.
- Repeated inflammatory cervical cytology.

Dyskaryosis or dysplasia on a cervical cytology sample refers to disproportionate nuclear enlargement in the cell in comparison to the amount of cytoplasm present. Dyskaryotic cells have abnormal chromatin content and distribution and may have abnormality in the nuclear shape.

Prior to the colposcopic examination, a relevant medical history should be obtained, ideally using a proforma designed specifically for the colposcopy clinic. Information should be obtained in relation to menstruation, contraception, pregnancies, smoking, previous cervical cytology, symptoms, previous treatments, and date of last menstrual period. A detailed explanation should be given to the patient with regards to the colposcopic examination. Written information should be given prior to the visit to the colposcopy department.

The colposcope is a binocular microscope that allows magnification and illumination of the cervix. By applying various stains to the cervix, abnormalities can be identified. These include benign, precancerous, and malignant changes. Its primary use is to evaluate abnormal cervical cytology as an aid to diagnosis. It can then be used to guide further management.

All colposcopes follow similar principles. They provide magnification between 6- and 40-fold. Low and

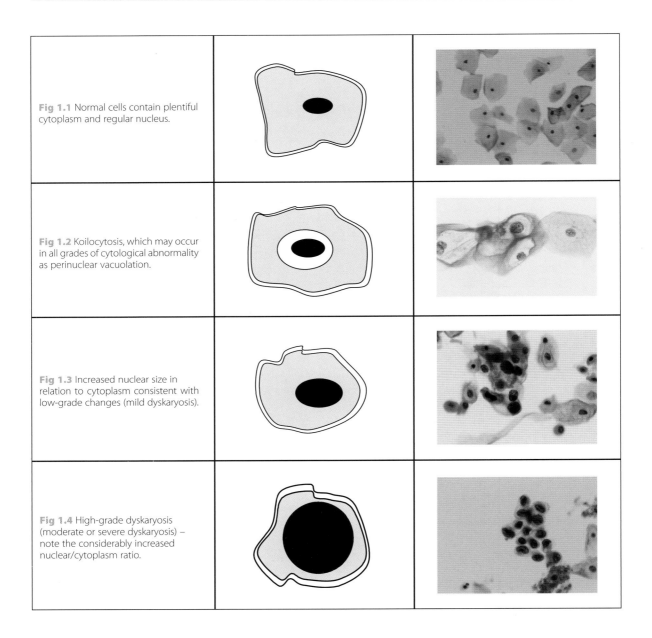

| | | |
|---|---|---|
| **Fig 1.1** Normal cells contain plentiful cytoplasm and regular nucleus. | | |
| **Fig 1.2** Koilocytosis, which may occur in all grades of cytological abnormality as perinuclear vacuolation. | | |
| **Fig 1.3** Increased nuclear size in relation to cytoplasm consistent with low-grade changes (mild dyskaryosis). | | |
| **Fig 1.4** High-grade dyskaryosis (moderate or severe dyskaryosis) – note the considerably increased nuclear/cytoplasm ratio. | | |

medium magnification is used for initial assessment; high magnification (20-fold plus) is used to detect the finer detail of vascular patterns. A green filter allows better visualisation of vasculature on the cervix.

Colposcopy is best carried out on days 10–14 of the menstrual cycle when the cervical mucus is clear and not tenacious. Colposcopic assessment is difficult when there is significant vaginal bleeding. If the woman is menstruating, the procedure should be postponed.

If the presenting symptoms were of vaginal bleeding in the presence of a suspicious looking cervix, then the woman should be seen irrespective of bleeding status to rule out the possibility of invasive disease. Common sense needs to prevail in scheduling the appointment. Women taking the oral contraceptive pill can continue with this to allow colposcopic assessment to take place for the convenience of the woman and the clinic.

# How to choose a colposcope

There are a variety of colposcopes available. Only by trialling some of these colposcopes will the correct decision be made in terms of choosing the right colposcopic equipment for your particular environment. Some of the criteria that should be assessed are:

- Cost – can vary considerably. Affordability is one of the most important factors in decision making.
- Optical quality – the better the optics, the better the colposcopic image. This relates to brightness, clarity, and an evenly illuminated image.
- Zoom magnification – there should be a good range of magnifications available. Most have a stepped magnification although some have a continuously variable mechanism.
- Design should allow the colposcopic arm to be counter-balanced to ensure smooth movement and stability in usage.
- Eyepiece – should feel comfortable in usage. Many have diopter adjustment for visual correction of myopia (short sightedness) and hypermetropia (long sightedness).
- Focal length – usually fixed, although in some may be variable to a degree, which allows the colposcopist to be optimally positioned for the procedure.
- Illumination – should have good even light with facility for green filter. The bulb should be easily changeable.
- Fixtures – can be free standing, wall, ceiling or chair mounted depending on the clinical environment. Size and maneuvrability may be important if the colposcope is to be used in more than one setting.
- Operating environment – make sure that colposcope will function given the clinic air temperature and humidity level.
- Optional accessories:
  - Display facilities – by attaching to a monitor, live images can be displayed for education and teaching functions. Otherwise a teaching arm is useful.
  - Recording facilities – documentation is becoming increasingly important and digital formats are ideal for this purpose. One can either use still or video formats.

# The following instruments should be available

- Examination gloves.
- Cervical sampling devices – cervical brushes (e.g. cytobrush, cervex brush), spatulae (e.g. Ayre's, Aylebury's, or plastic spatula).
- Container for liquid-based cytology; glass slides (plus fixative) for traditional cytology.
- Bivalve speculum of varying size and lubricant.
- Three small pots containing saline, acetic acid (3–5%), and Lugol's iodine.
- Cotton wool balls.
- Sponge holding forceps.
- Cotton-tip and jumbo swabs.
- Endocervical canal specula.
- Biopsy forceps and pots with fixative for specimens.
- Haemostatic solutions/substances – e.g. monsel's solution (ferrous subsulphate) dried to a thick paste or silver nitrate sticks.

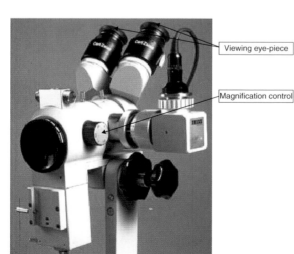

**Fig 1.5** Colposcope.

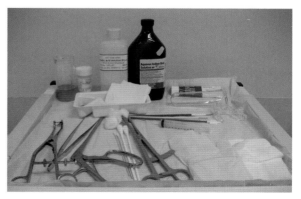

**Fig 1.6** Colposcopy trolley.

## Technique of colposcopy

Patients should be examined in warm relaxed surroundings having been fully informed about the procedure. The woman is helped onto the couch in the lithotomy position. Leg supports should be comfortable and the couch adjusted appropriately. External genitalia should be assessed for any obvious abnormalities. A suitably sized speculum is used to expose the cervix. If the vaginal sidewalls obstruct the view, they can be displaced by using the finger of an examination glove (or a condom) placed over the speculum blades.

If required a cervical cytology sample is taken but if the woman is presenting with cytological

abnormality, this should be avoided as it can cause unnecessary bleeding and interference with the colposcopic examination. A variety of sampling devices are available.

Liquid-based cytology relies on the sampler being either immersed or agitated in fixative fluid (rinse using a vigorous swirling motion and then push the brush into the bottom of the vial at least ten times forcing the bristles apart). The cervical brushes are ideal for this purpose because some of these have detachable ends. Certain plastic spatulas also have detachable ends for this purpose. To obtain the cytology sample, the Cervex brush is rotated clockwise five times after being applied to the cervix. Where sampling of the endocervix is important, then a cytobrush should be used additionally. If a Papanicolaou smear (Pap smear) is required, then this may be obtained by the use of wooden/plastic spatulae or cervical brushes.

If a cervical cytology sample is required, this should be taken before the application of acetic acid. Occasionally, if one forgets and acetic acid is applied before taking the cervical sample, then this should be annotated on the cytology request form.

The cervix and upper vagina are examined at low magnification. Any excess mucus or blood should be removed using a dry or saline-soaked cotton wool ball. Presence of gross lesions and leukoplakia should be identified. The green filter should be used to assess the vascular pattern (low to high power). Benign lesions

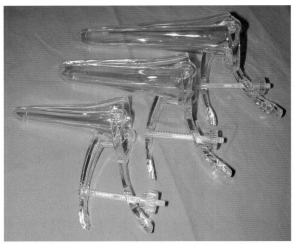

**Fig 1.7** Variety of speculae in large, medium, and small size. Bivalve with screw and lever for opening speculum.

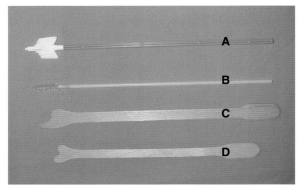

**Fig 1.8** Various sampling devices for taking cervical cytology – cervex brush (A), cytobrush (B), Aylesbury spatula (C), Ayres spatula (D).

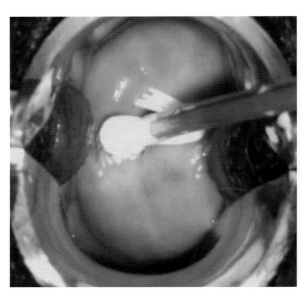

**Fig 1.9** Cervex brush being used for cytology sample taking.

that are visualized should be noted. These include Nabothian follicles, cervical polyps, warts, cysts etc.

Acetic acid (3–5%) is gently applied to the cervix with saturated cotton wool balls on sponge forceps or a jumbo swab, or by using a spray or syringe. Unnecessary abrasion should be avoided. The acetic acid is left in contact with the cervix for 10 seconds.

Following acetic acid application, any remaining mucus may be removed easily. Further acetic acid is applied as necessary. The cervical landmarks and any atypical areas should be mentally mapped. If image recording facilities are available, then these should be used liberally and stored either digitally or in print format. Lugol's iodine (1% iodine, 2% potassium iodide, 97% distilled water) may be used to further delineate atypical epithelium that contains little or no glycogen and therefore fails to take up the iodine stain. Normal squamous epithelium turns mahogany brown with Lugol's iodine. Columnar epithelium also contains little or no glycogen and fails to take up the stain. This is referred to as 'Schiller's test'. A positive Schiller's test refers to non-staining (i.e. iodine negative) and vice versa. Any excess solutions are removed from the vagina prior to removal of the speculum. The vagina should be examined as the speculum is removed. Immediately following assessment, the findings are recorded, ideally in a standard format.

- Was the squamocolumnar junction visible?
- Was there any acetowhite epithelium? If yes, document its site and size in graphic format (see Chapters 2 and 4).
- Assess the degree of change (see Chapter 4).

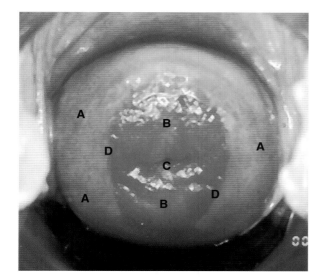

**Fig 1.10** Normal cervix with ectropion squamous epithelium (A) surrounds columnar epithelium (B) and cervical canal (C). Junction between the two types of epithelia is the SCJ (D).

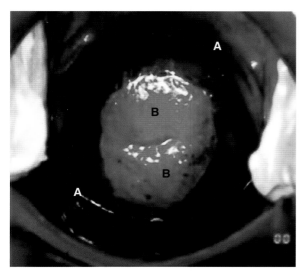

**Fig 1.11** Normal cervix with application of Lugol's iodine. Columnar epithelium (B) with minimal stain surrounded by glycogenated normal squamous epithelium (A), which stains darkly.

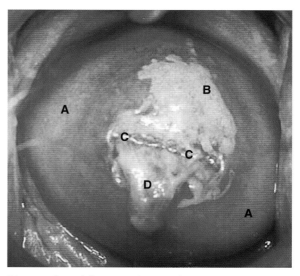

**Fig 1.12** Cervix following application of acetic acid. Squamous epithelium (A), acetowhite changes with sharp border (B), cervical canal and SCJ (C), cervical mucus – viscid following acetic acid application (D).

5

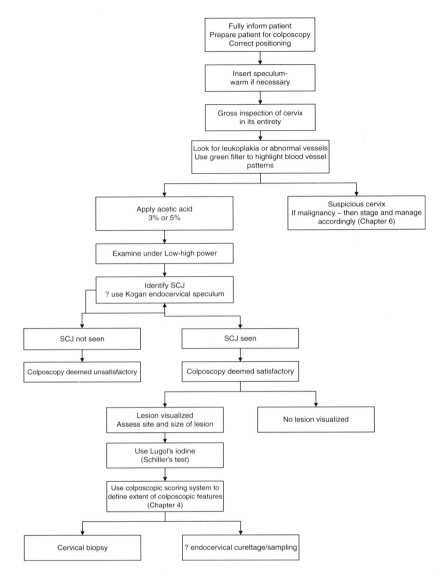

**Fig 1.13** Colposcopy flowchart.

## Learning points

- Colposcopy is appropriate in women with cytological abnormality.
- Women attending for colposcopy should be adequately informed and counseled.
- Dedicated facilities for colposcopy are ideal with appropriate back-up facilities.
- There needs to be good communication channels between the cytology, colposcopy, and histopathology services.
- Saline, acetic acid, and Lugol's iodine are used sequentially and changes on the cervix noted.
- Accurate documentation is necessary and this can be facilitated with the use of a proforma.
- Digital image storage is recommended or other form of image capture.

# Chapter 2

# The normal cervix and colposcopic appearance

A detailed knowledge of the normal appearance of the cervix is important prior to looking for colposcopic abnormalities. The size and shape of the cervix shows considerable variation amongst individuals and at different stages of an individual's life. Puberty and pregnancy in particular have significant effects on the cervix. Menopause may cause atrophic changes, which may lead to specific changes that may cause difficulties with screening and colposcopy.

In the adult, the cervix measures 2.5–3 cm in length. In the nulliparous, the external cervical os is circular whereas the multiparous cervix is slit-like in the transverse dimension. The cervix contains two types of epithelia, the stratified squamous, which lines the vaginal portion (ectocervix), and the simple columnar lining the cervical canal (endocervix), which is flattened in the anteroposterior dimension.

The understanding of the appearance and the relationship of the different epithelia types is described.

## Squamous epithelium

Two types of squamous epithelia may be present – original or transformed. The original squamous epithelium is a featureless smooth, pink epithelium originally established on the cervix and vagina. Squamous epithelium is similar to that found in the rest of the vagina and is multilayered. The epithelium does not stain white after the application of a dilute solution of acetic acid and stains brown after the application of Lugol's iodine.

In the transformed squamous epithelium, gland openings may be visualized on colposcopic assessment. If these gland openings become blocked for various reasons, then Nabothian follicles could be present.

## Columnar epithelium

Columnar epithelium is a single-layer, mucus-producing epithelium that extends between the endometrium cranially and either the original squamous epithelium or the metaplastic (transformed) squamous epithelium caudally. Columnar epithelium is normally present in the endocervix and may be present on the ectocervix (ectopy) or, on rare occasions, in the vagina. The epithelium appears red and velvety, contrasting with the pink squamous epithelium. Each villi that

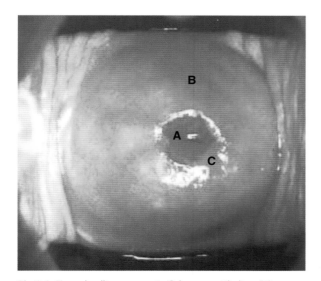

**Fig 2.1** Normal nulliparous cervix. Columnar epithelium (A) surrounded by squamous epithelium (B). Border between two epithelial types is the SCJ (C).

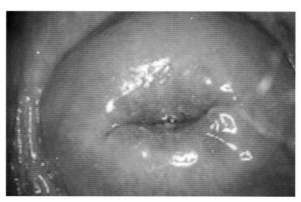

**Fig 2.2** Normal cervix in parous woman. Cervical os appears slit-like.

gives it a characteristic appearance has a central blood supply.

At colposcopy the area has a typical grape-like structure. Application of acetic acid causes columnar epithelium to turn white and the villi become less distinct. As the epithelium is thin with blood vessels just below, contact bleeding may occur.

## Squamocolumnar junction

The squamocolumnar junction (SCJ) of the cervix is defined as the border between the stratified squamous epithelium and the mucin-secreting columnar epithelium of the endocervix. Two types of SCJ are described:

> The *original* SCJ – site where the native squamous and columnar epithelia meet each other. This is present from birth. The exact location of the SCJ varies between individuals and at various stages in an individual's life.

At the time of menarche, both the cervix and uterus enlarge. This enlargement causes an eversion of the cervix so that more of the columnar epithelium is visible on the vaginal surface of the cervix. As the environment in the vagina is different from the endocervix, especially high acidity, the epithelium undergoes a process of transformation – metaplasia – and eventually is replaced by the stratified multilayered squamous epithelium. This gives rise to an acquired or *new* SCJ.

The *new* SCJ is at the junction of the metaplastic area and the columnar epithelium. This is an important landmark and is relevant for the full assessment of the transformation zone (TZ).

## Metaplasia

This is the physiological replacement of one type of mature epithelium by another equally mature type of epithelium. In the cervix, squamous metaplasia is the replacement of the mucin-secreting columnar epithelium by a stratified squamous epithelium. Varying stages from immature to mature metaplasia may be recognized on colposcopic assessment. The metaplastic process is irreversible and maximal during times of high estrogenic stimulation. These occur mainly during adolescence, whilst taking the combined oral contraceptive, and during the first pregnancy. It is important not to confuse the immature metaplastic process with abnormality.

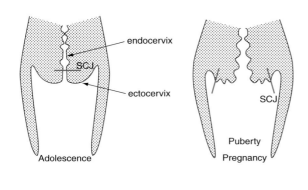
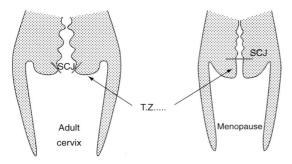

**Fig 2.3** The apparent migration of the SCJ secondary to hormonal influence.

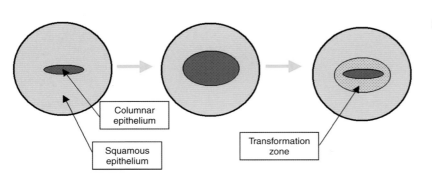

**Fig 2.4** Process of metaplasia.

Colposcopic features suggestive of metaplastic change:

- Smooth surface with fine, uniform-caliber vessels
- Mild acetowhite change
- Negative or partial positivity with Lugol's iodine

## The transformation zone

The transformation zone (TZ) is the area between the original squamous and columnar epithelium within which varying degrees of maturity may be identified. The TZ is of variable shape and size. At different stages of maturity the metaplastic epithelium may stain slightly white after the application of acetic acid and partially brown after the application of Lugol's iodine. Components of a normal TZ may be islands of columnar epithelium surrounded by metaplastic squamous epithelium, cleft openings and Nabothian cysts.

There are three types of TZ:

- A type 1 TZ is completely ectocervical and fully visible, and may be small or large.
- A type 2 TZ has an endocervical component, is fully visible, and may have an ectocervical component that may be small or large.
- A type 3 TZ has an endocervical component that is not fully visible and may have an ectocervical component that may be small or large.

In a small percentage of women the TZ may extend caudally onto the upper vagina, usually with an anterior and posterior triangle or tongue; it may contain a fine regular mosaic pattern of blood vessels and stain partially or wholly negative after the application of Lugol's iodine.

## Ectropion

This relates to the eversion of the columnar epithelium so that it is visible in the vaginal portion of the cervix. Although a physiological phenomenon, it can cause confusion in colposcopic assessment, especially if large and fragile. Ectropions can cause symptoms of vaginal discharge (excess mucin secretion) or postcoital bleeding (contact bleeding from fragile thin columnar epithelium). Cervical ectropion does not warrant any treatment unless there are related symptoms. Before undertaking treatment it is advisable to rule out an infectious cause such as chlamydia. If ablative treatment is undertaken, it is important to have a normal cervical cytology history and even biopsy if there is clinical suspicion. Cryocautery is the commonest method of treating ectropion as it can be conducted in clinic without recourse to anesthesia and has relatively high success rates. An alternative method is diathermy ablation for which local anesthesia is recommended. If necessary, treatment can be repeated in those with continuing symptoms.

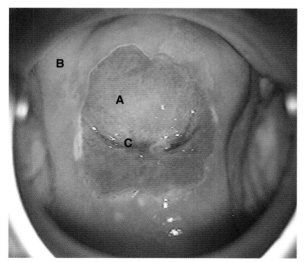

**Fig 2.5** Normal cervix with cervical ectropion. Columnar epithelium (A) and squamous epithelium (B), cervical canal (C).

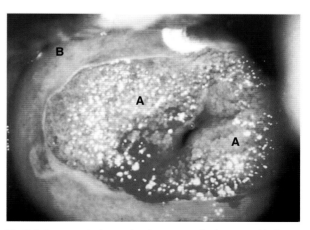

**Fig 2.6** Large cervical ectropion. Large area of columnar epithelium (A) exposed and surrounded by squamous epithelium (B).

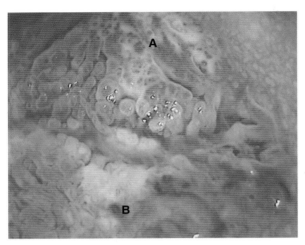

**Fig 2.7** Metaplastic changes (A) within the TZ. Gland openings (B).

## Pathophysiology at different stages in a woman's life

At birth, most females will have some degree of mucin-secreting columnar epithelium present on the vaginal portion of the cervix. At about one year of age, the cervix begins to elongate and causes the SCJ to move towards the external os.

After menarche, a cervical ectropion is present by the eversion of the columnar epithelium onto the vaginal portion of the cervix. This undergoes physiologic metaplasia to squamous epithelium. These changes are maximal under the age of 20 and during first pregnancy.

At the menopause, there is inversion of the cervix. This makes access to the TZ difficult. Cervical cytology and colposcopy is more likely to be unsatisfactory as the area of concern may be within the endocervix to varying degrees. A short course of estrogen may reverse these changes allowing better cytological and colposcopic assessment.

## Learning points

- Recognition of normality and its variations is important for colposcopy.
- The cervix is dynamic, undergoing changes from fetus until old age.
- Metaplasia and the replacement of columnar by squamous epithelium is a normal, irreversible, physiological process.
- Sampling from the TZ by cytology and its assessment by colposcopy varies according to the age of the woman.
- Columnar epithelium is single layered and allows visualization of vasculature beneath the epithelium (appears red).
- Squamous epithelium is multilayered and appears pink on examination.
- Recognition of the TZ and its varying stages of metaplasia is important for colposcopic practice.

# Natural history of cervical carcinoma, HPV, and vaccination

Cervical cancer is the third commonest female cancer worldwide, with breast and colorectal cancer occurring more often. It accounts for 10% of the cancers in women worldwide and is the most commonly diagnosed cancer among women in Southern Africa and Central America. There is a seven-fold variation in the incidence of cervical cancer between the different regions of the world. Cervical cancer is potentially the most preventable major form of cancer, given the prolonged phased natural history of precancerous stage. Those countries that have introduced organized cervical screening programs have seen significant falls in the incidence and mortality associated with cervical cancer. Coverage rates of the at-risk population need to be high (>80%) in order to achieve the desired effect; however, a much greater effect on control of this disease in these countries was achieved even prior to introduction of formal screening programs. This was attributable to health education and empowerment of women leading to increased awareness amongst populations, regular check-ups and availability of appropriate management services. In developing countries,

similar efforts could help bring down the high rates of cervical cancer by devoting more resources to educational programs.

Within Europe there is a variation in incidence of cervical cancer depending on the availability and implementation of the cervical screening and management program. Across Europe, cervical cancer is the fifth most common cancer in women. In the UK, cervical cancer is now the eleventh most common cancer in women and accounts for 2% of all female cancers. The estimated lifetime risk of a female developing cervical cancer is 1 in 136 in the UK.

There are many risk factors associated with cervical cancer but many of these are surrogates for sexual activity. The risk factors include:

- Human papilloma virus (HPV) infection – recognizably the most important etiological risk factor. Evidence linking HPV with cervical cancer is extremely strong and satisfies virtually all the epidemiological criteria for causality – namely strength, consistency and specificity of

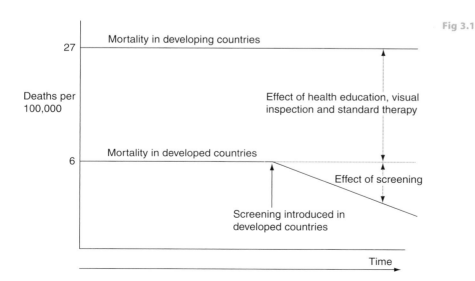

Fig 3.1

association, temporality of events, biological gradient, plausibility, and experimental evidence. Whilst exposure is important, it is the persistence of HPV that is related to the development of CIN and invasive cervical disease (see below).

- Early onset of sexual activity – generally taken as age 16 or younger.
- Multiple sexual partners (self or of the partner) – this relates to the exposure to high-risk oncogenic HPV. The prevalence of HPV approaches 100% in women involved in unprotected sex with multiple partners.
- Low socioeconomic status – this may relate to many other factors that are inter-related; however, it has been shown that women from a low socioeconomic social class have three times increased risk of developing cervical cancer, irrespective of other associated risk factors.
- Tobacco smoking – there is evidence that smoking increases risk of invasive cervical cancer and also interacts with HPV in carcinogenic effect. The increased risk for smokers is around two-fold, with the highest risk in those with long-term and high-intensity use. Smoking does not appear to be associated with increased risk for adenocarcinoma.
- Use of oral contraceptive pill – a long-term follow-up study of women using oral contraceptive pill found a relative risk of death from cervical cancer of 2.5 among current and recent users (within 10 years) compared to never users. A three-fold increased risk for invasive squamous cell cervical cancer was found for women who were HPV positive and had used oral contraception for five or more years.
- Other sexually transmitted infections – namely, herpes simplex virus, Chlamydia, and bacterial vaginosis. No direct causal link has been established with any of these infections; however, evidence is emerging suggesting a catalytic role of these agents with HPV in progression of dysplastic changes.
- Immunocompromise – organ transplant patients, Lupus disease and human immunodeficiency virus (HIV) infection. In these women the increased risk may be five-fold. Treatment for HIV infection will ameliorate its effect. All these women are also at

higher risk of residual/recurrent disease after treatment.
- Malnutrition – the weight of evidence, albeit inconclusive, from several contradictory studies indicates that consumption of fruit and vegetables and some associated micronutrients (beta-carotene, vitamin C, and folate) are protective against invasive cancer.
- Multiparity – again a controversial role. Multiparity may be indicative of sexual activity and tissue damage rather than having direct causative role.

## Natural history

It has been estimated that the mean time from detectable cytologic abnormality to development of invasive cancer may take as long as 15–20 years. Thus, progression of CIN to invasive cancer, although it can be swift, is usually a slow process.

Many CIN lesions will regress over time. The regression rate depends, amongst other factors, mainly upon the grade of CIN and the age of the woman. Regression is much more common in women under 30 years than those above 30 years of age. Taken together, in the absence of intervention, roughly one-third of early precursor lesions disappear spontaneously, one-third persist, and one-third progress to CIN III or invasive cancer.

The progressive potential of cervical intraepithelial neoplasia varies according to grade of abnormality. In high-grade lesions (CIN II & III), the lesions have definite progressive potential that can be lowered dramatically by treatment of this precancerous phase. In those that are treated, even though their cervical cytology may revert to normal, they remain at increased risk for the development of invasive cervical cancer compared to the general population without cytological abnormality. In those women with abnormal cervical cytology following treatment for CIN, the risk is 25–30 times the background rate for the development of cervical cancer. Women with lesser abnormalities such as CIN I have an unknown but low malignant risk. Management of women with these disorders depends on other variables such as age and compliance to cytological surveillance programs. Women who are immunocompromised are at particular risk for the progression of preinvasive lesions to the malignant phase.

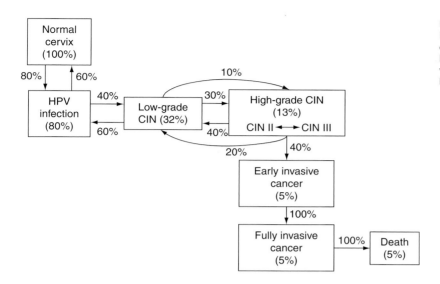

**Fig 3.2** Flow representation of natural history of CIN – the percentages given are estimates of what might happen over a lifetime in the absence of screening, vaccination, and treatment (adapted from P Sasieni, Cancer Research, UK).

In those women with hrHPV infection, they are more likely to develop preinvasive disease and then develop the invasive form. Most of the HPV infections are transient, about 60–80%, depending on the age, clear spontaneously within 1–2 years. The rest would result in CIN lesions. Most of the women with HPV positive cytology who develop CIN lesions are still able to clear the virus in 2–3 years and will subsequently have regressive CIN; however, above 30 years the regression rate is much lower. Among women with persistent infection, CIN lesions can develop within 2–4 years. The progression rate of CIN in women with hrHPV positive test, cytologically normal or abnormal cervical sample is about 5% per year. In women above 30 years with positive hrHPV, cytologically normal cervical sample the risk of developing CIN III is 116 times higher than women with a negative hrHPV cytologically normal cervical sample.

## Determinants of disease progression or regression

The development of minor cervical cytological abnormality is common in young women. The majority of these will be a transient phase and will regress back to normal over time. Most of the risk factors listed earlier are potential determinants of progression rather than prime etiological agents. Those women with persistent high-risk oncogenic HPV infection and those with repeated exposure to infections remain at risk for disease progression. Women who are exposed to tobacco smoking are more likely to have disease persistence or progression compared to non-smokers or those that cease smoking. Women who are immunocompromised are likewise more likely to have disease progression. It has been established that the age of the host, >30 years, is an independent determinant of oncogenic progression.

The size of lesion and grade of abnormality is related to malignant potential. High-grade intraepithelial disease and large lesions have significantly higher malignant potential compared with low-grade and small lesions. The tumor biology may vary and different cancer types will have a different natural history.

## Human papilloma virus

Whilst HPV is present in virtually all cervical tumors, most HPV infections will not progress to CIN or cancer. The invasive disease does not develop unless there is persistence of HPV deoxyribonucleic acid (DNA) and it has been proposed as the first ever identified 'necessary cause' of a human cancer. Out of the >150 known HPV genotypes, 30 are known to infect the genital tract. Out of these, 20 have been identified as carcinogenic with types 16 and 18 found most commonly in malignant lesions.

The common types are classified according to their oncogenic potential as follows:

Low risk: 6, 11, 26, 40, 42, 53, 54, 55, 57, 66, 73, 82, 83, 84

High risk: 16, 18, 31, 33, 35, 39, 45, 51, 52, 56, 58, 59, 66, 68, 73, 82

Both high- and low-risk HPV infections in women occur mostly in adolescent age groups (16–24 years). Reported incidences from different countries have been 10–30%. The incidence drops to about 5% above the age of 30 years. Most of these HPV infections are transient and clear spontaneously within 1–2 years.

Testing for the hrHPV types is becoming clinical practice in the triage of minor cytological abnormalities (borderline/ASC-US and mild dyskaryosis/LSIL). A number of different diagnostic kits are available that test for the hrHPV types using differing technologies including some that are able to genotype. These hrHPV tests can be performed either serially or as co-testing with cervical cytology. The consistency of tests for hrHPV is higher when compared with cytology. It also has clinical applicability in 'test of cure' following treatment for CIN. Testing for HPV in the primary screening setting is being actively studied where it can detect prevalent disease as well as predict risk.

## HPV vaccination

HPV is a necessary cause for cervical cancer. It is additionally associated with other genital tract cancers including the vagina, vulva, anus, penis, as well as oropharynx and tonsils. HPV 16 is the main causative agent at these various sites, with other oncogenic types contributing particularly to cervical cancer risk. HPV enters the basal layer through microabrasions at the surface of the epithelium. In approximately 90%, HPV clearance occurs within three years of infection. When there is viral persistence, then precancerous and cancerous changes can occur. The natural antibody response is mainly type-specific as compared to the cross-protection achieved with vaccination.

The currently available vaccines (Gardasil® and Cervarix®) consist of virus-like particles (VLPs) of HPV 16 and 18 that together cause about 70% of the worldwide occurring cases of cervical cancer. Gardasil contains, in addition, VLPs of HPV types 6 and 11 that induce the majority (90%) of genital warts. Both vaccines have an excellent safety profile. There are ongoing studies looking at using a vaccine with nine HPV types, seven of which are oncogenic.

## Currently available HPV vaccines

| | Quadrivalent vaccine | Bivalent vaccine |
|---|---|---|
| Manufacturer & trade name | Merck, Gardasil® | GlaxoSmithKline, Cervarix® |
| HPV genotypes | 6, 11, 16, 18 | 16, 18 |
| Adjuvant | Proprietary Aluminum | Proprietary Aluminum plus Monophosphoryl Lipid A |
| Schedule: 3 IM doses at | 0, 2, 6 months | 0, 1, 6 months |
| Age range | 9–26 27–45 (FDA) | 10–25 recommended >10 |

The current vaccines do not provide a therapeutic effect against prevalent infections hence vaccination is most cost-effective when given before exposure, i.e. before the sexual debut. In the UK, this is offered to girls aged 12–13 through the schools. Unlike natural exposure, HPV vaccination invariably induces seroconversion with noticeably far higher titers of antibody levels. These antibody levels remain high for at least 10 years, which is the current duration of study. It is likely that the protection will remain high for much longer, but these long-term studies are ongoing.

A reduction of cervical cancer rates may only be expected in 20–30 years, but a 25% decrease in abnormal cervical cytology tests in women aged <30 and associated colposcopy referral may be expected within a few years, just as an up to 70% diminishment in excisional treatments for high-grade disease. Furthermore, additional gain can be expected from a reduction of vulvar, vaginal, and anal cancers and their precursors, which are also partly caused by HPV 16 and 18. There will also be a beneficial effect on the incidence of oropharyngeal and oral cavity cancers as the immunity is systemic. For the benefit to be maximized, there is a need for high coverage of the at risk population (80% or greater). Vaccinated women should still attend cervical screening programs, otherwise the incidence of cervical cancer could even double since up to 30% of all cervical cancer cases are caused by non-vaccine types.

## Learning points

- There are multiple risk factors for cervical cancers, many of these being surrogates for sexual activity.
- The process of cervical cancer development is generally slow, allowing screening to take place and intervention to alter the natural history.
- Non-invasive changes on the cervix may change over time, allowing for conservative management approaches in certain situations.
- Persistence of high-risk oncogenic HPV infection appears to be important for the pathogenesis of cervical cancer.

- Education and general healthcare provision has a significant impact on the incidence of cervical cancer.
- Countries with planned population-based screening programs have seen the largest effect on cervical cancer incidence and mortality.
- HPV vaccination is available, which provides protection against cervical intraepithelial neoplasia (and anticipated protection against cervical cancer).
- The HPV vaccine has beneficial protection against other anogenital and oropharyngeal cancers.

# Chapter 4

# Colposcopic appearance of CIN

Assessment of women presenting with abnormal cervical cytology and the selection of those requiring treatment relies on colposcopic assessment of the cervical TZ. Colposcopy remains subjective, and expertise in recognizing differing patterns and their corresponding histological abnormalities is dependent upon a period of apprenticeship. Differentiation of normal and abnormal colposcopic findings and their relative importance is of great significance in the management of women with abnormal cervical cytology or those suspected of invasive disease. Recognizing what is normal is an essential prerequisite before being able to recognize abnormality.

The two sites of possible colposcopic abnormality reside within the epithelia and the vasculature of the cervix, therefore knowledge of the appearances of the three types of normal epithelia and their relationship is of considerable importance. These epithelia are:

- Squamous
- Columnar
- Metaplastic

The TZ is variable in width and configuration and contains columnar and squamous metaplastic epithelium of varying maturity. The use of the green filter aids the recognition of vascular patterns.

## Atypical transformation zone

The atypical transformation zone (ATZ) is the area of the cervix whose limits define cervical intraepithelial neoplasia. The TZ is a dynamic region of the epithelium and deviation to abnormality occurs within the unstable metaplastic epithelium; however, there is no one feature that defines a distinct histological abnormality and it is the overall appearance that is important. Any condition that causes increased cellular division, abnormal cellular metabolism, or increased vascularisation can produce atypical colposcopic findings in cervical epithelium.

There are various characteristics of the ATZ and these will be discussed individually. Scoring systems in common usage will be discussed as well as a clinico–colposcopic index (CCI) that takes into account the patient characteristics as well as known prognostic colposcopic factors to predict the degree of abnormality of the TZ.

## Cytological and histological parameters (nomenclature) of CIN

The original cytological classification introduced by Papanicolaou has been largely replaced worldwide. The currently used cytological terminology in the UK was proposed by the British Society for Clinical Cytology in 1987, where the appearances of the cells are classified into mild, moderate, and severe dyskaryosis, with borderline nuclear abnormalities used for changes that fall short of dyskaryosis. 'Severe dyskaryosis ?invasive disease' may be used as may '?glandular neoplasia' in those cases where the dyskaryosis appears to be in glandular cells. The National Cancer Institute of the United States developed The Bethesda system (TBS) in 1988, which was modified in 2001. This classifies abnormalities as atypical squamous or glandular cells of undetermined significance (ASC-US), atypical squamous cells but cannot exclude HSIL (ASC-H), low grade squamous intraepithelial lesions, LSIL (encompassing HPV and CIN I) and high-grade squamous intraepithelial lesions, HSIL (encompassing CIN II and CIN III). The various abnormalities can co-exist but management is dictated by the worst histological diagnosis. Irrespective of the terminology used, there is debate as to whether CIN is a continuum.

The histogenetic classification of cervical precancerous lesions, which reflects the depth of epithelial involvement, was first introduced by the World Health Organization (WHO). In 1967, CIN classification was

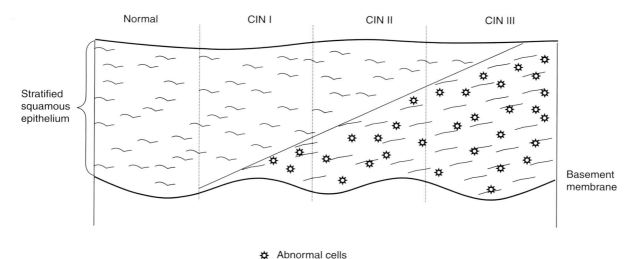

**Fig 4.1** CIN is graded on the proportion of epithelium containing abnormal cells (original by G Teale, Australia).

introduced by Richart where CIN I, II, and III corresponds to mild, moderate and severe dysplasia/carcinoma in situ (CIS) of WHO classification, respectively. In 1990 a revised classification was suggested by Richart, with high-grade lesions (CIN II/III) likely to be true cancer precursors and low-grade lesions (CIN I / HPV) with unknown or low progressive potential. In actual practice the WHO and the three-tier CIN classifications are used universally.

## Colposcopic parameters and their relative importance

An important element of colposcopy is to view the cervix prior to application of acetic acid. This can be aided by gently cleansing the area with saline and using the green filter to accentuate any vascular patterns. Epithelial alterations to note are leukoplakia and acetowhite epithelium. The vascular changes include punctation, mosaic, and atypical vessels.

## Leukoplakia

Leukoplakia is visible without application of acetic acid even to the naked eye. It appears as a white area of thickened epithelium, which maybe patchy or cover large areas of cervix and sometimes extends onto the vagina. Histologically it denotes hyperkeratosis or parakeratosis. Its main significance is that it may obscure visualization of the TZ. Biopsy should always be done.

## Acetowhite epithelium

After the application of a dilute solution of 3–5% acetic acid, areas of high nuclear density appear white. Although this may occur in cases of immature metaplasia, generally the denser the acetowhite change, the faster the change becomes apparent, and the increased length of time the epithelium holds the change, the more severe the lesion may be. Dense acetowhite change within columnar epithelium may indicate glandular disease.

Acetowhite epithelium is not diagnostic for CIN. Other conditions that display acetowhiteness are:

- HPV related changes
- Mixture of CIN and HPV
- Columnar epithelium
- Immature squamous metaplasia
- Healing or regenerating epithelium
- Congenital TZ
- Inflammation
- Adenocarcinoma in situ or Adenocarcinoma
- Invasive squamous cell carcinoma (SCC)

In general the more intense and sustained the acetowhite change, the more significant the lesion. The margins may be well defined but appear indistinct or fuzzy, particularly with HPV-related lesions. The size of the lesion can be a good predictor of histological grade of the precancerous lesion. This can either be assessed by the number of quadrants involved with acetowhite change or by the lesion surface area. A large lesion

**17**

## Classification systems of cervical intraepithelial neoplasia compared

| CIN classification | WHO classification | The Bethesda System classification* | Squamous intraepithelial neoplasia (SIL) classification | Histology |
|---|---|---|---|---|
| CIN I | Mild dysplasia | Low-grade CIN | Low-grade SIL (LSIL) | Abnormal cells occupy basal third of the epithelium |
| | | | |  Fig 4.2 |
| CIN II | Moderate dysplasia | High-grade CIN | High-grade SIL (HSIL) | Abnormal cells occupy 1/3–2/3 of epithelium |
| | | | |  Fig 4.3 |
| CIN III | Severe dysplasia / carcinoma in situ | High-grade CIN | High-grade SIL (HSIL) | Abnormal cells occupy >2/3 of epithelium |
| | | | |  Fig 4.4 |

*Within The Bethesda System Classification, low-grade CIN incorporates wart virus infection.

would be greater than 1 cm². Despite the correlation of histological grade of CIN with lesion size, CIN III may occur as a small focus and CIN I may be extensive.

## Iodine negativity

After the application of Lugol's iodine, mature squamous epithelium, which contains glycogen, will stain a deep brown. Iodine-negative areas may represent immature metaplasia, cervical intraepithelial neoplasia, or low estrogen states (i.e. atrophy). A speckled appearance in an area with slight acetowhite change may represent immature metaplasia or low-grade intraepithelial neoplasia. Complete iodine negativity, a yellow staining in an area that has appeared strongly

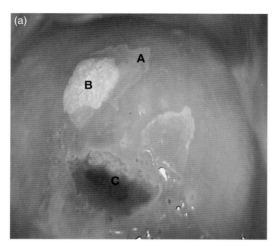

Fig 4.5a Low-grade CIN (A), HPV lesion (B), cervical canal (C).

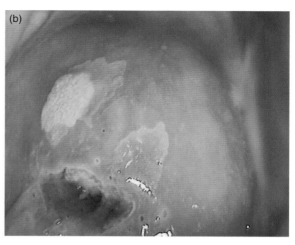

Fig 4.5b Same lesion as in 4.5(a) but with green filter applied.

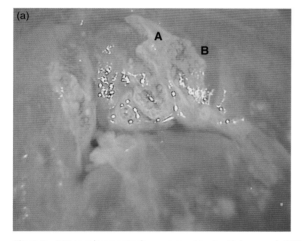

Fig 4.6a Minor colposcopic changes consistent with low-grade CIN (A). Border between atypical area and normal squamous epithelium is fairly indistinct (B).

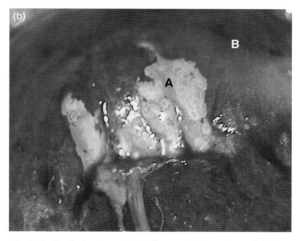

Fig 4.6b Similar lesion as 4.6(a) after application of Lugol's iodine. Atycical area (A)fails to stain and is termed schiller's test posivive. Normal squamous epithelium stains a dark brown color (B).

acetowhite, is highly suggestive of high-grade intraepithelial neoplasia. The use of Lugol's iodine is useful particularly for the beginner in delineating any abnormalities.

## Vascular patterns

The three identifiable vascular patterns are:

- *Mosaic*
  A focal colposcopic appearance in which the new vessel formation appears as a rectangular pattern like a mosaic. The smaller the mosaic, the more likely the lesion is to be of low grade or metaplasia.

The coarser, wider, and more irregular the mosaic, the more likely the lesion is to be of higher grade.

Often referred to as 'crazy-paving' pattern when the capillaries are seen parallel to the surface. In its minimal form it shows fine caliber vessels surrounding small areas of regular size and shape. In its maximal development the mosaic shows coarser, more hyperemic, more superficial vessels surrounding irregular fields, so that the intercapillary distance is increased. Often combinations of mosaic and punctation patterns intermingle.

- *Punctation*
  A focal colposcopic pattern in which capillaries appear in a stippled pattern. The finer the punctation

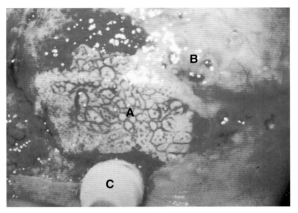

**Fig 4.7** CIN II with mosaic. Mosaic and punctation of various coarseness (A), gland opening (B), cotton bud manipulating cervix (C).

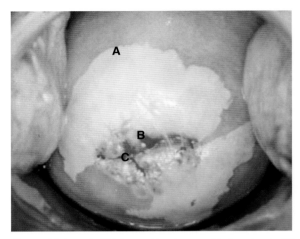

**Fig 4.8** High-grade CIN. Acetowhite change with sharp border (A), SCJ (B), cervical canal (C)

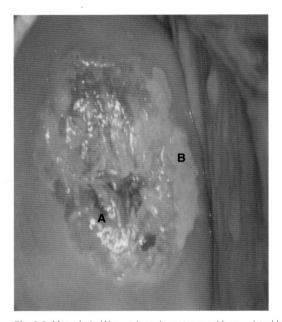

**Fig 4.9** Metaplasia (A) seen in various stages with associated high-grade CIN (B).

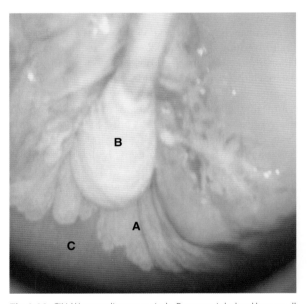

**Fig 4.10** CIN (A) extending posteriorly. Exposure is helped by a small cotton-tipped swab (B) with normal squamous epithelium (C) at periphery of cervix.

appearance, the more likely the lesion is to be of low grade or metaplasia. The coarser the punctation, the more likely the lesion is to be of higher grade.

Basic unit of the punctation pattern is the single, looped capillary within the stromal papilla, coursing obliquely or perpendicularly towards the surface of the epithelium, seen end-on as a dot. In its minimal development it is fine with closely spaced capillaries of narrow caliber forming regular patterns. Higher degrees of abnormality display capillaries with increased caliber and irregular spacing, even-coiled (corkscrew) vessels.

- *Atypical vessels*
  A focal abnormal colposcopic pattern in which the blood vessel pattern appears not as punctation or mosaic or as the finely branching capillaries of a normal epithelium, but rather as irregular vessels with an abrupt and interrupted course appearing as commas, corkscrew capillaries, or spaghetti-like

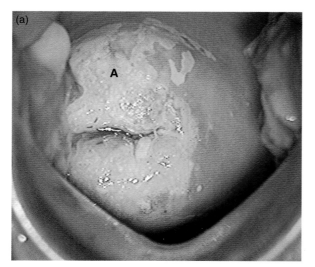

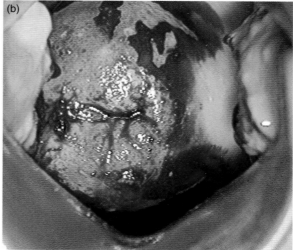

Fig 4.11 High-grade CIN (A) with acetic acid application and following Lugol's iodine application.

forms. Lesions, especially those with invasive changes, have new vessels that are formed often demonstrating gross variation in caliber, branching and arrangement. The intercapillary distance is much greater than is found in normal epithelium.

## Colposcopic features suggestive of low-grade disease (minor change)

- A smooth surface with an irregular outer border.
- Slight acetowhite change, slow to appear, and quick to disappear.
- Mild, often speckled iodine partial positivity.
- Fine punctation and fine regular mosaic.

## Colposcopic features suggestive of high-grade disease (major change)

- A generally smooth surface with a sharp outer border.
- Dense acetowhite change, that appears early and is slow to resolve; it may be oyster white.
- Iodine negativity, a yellow appearance in a previously dense white epithelium.
- Coarse punctation and wide irregular mosaics of differing size.
- Dense acetowhite change within columnar epithelium may indicate glandular disease.

## Colposcopic features suggestive of invasive cancer

- Irregular surface, erosion, or ulceration.
- Dense acetowhite change.
- Wide irregular punctation and mosaic.
- Atypical vessels.

## Grading systems

A variety of formal grading schemes have been suggested. All of these are dependent upon a subjective assessment of the colposcopic features. Any grading system should be simple to use and practical in a clinical setting. With adequate training and a systematic approach to colposcopic assessment, it is possible to categorize many lesions affecting the cervix and thereby differentiate between significant as opposed to insignificant lesions.

One of these grading systems analysed data collected prospectively. Of the clinical variables, the referral cervical cytology and smoking status were statistically the most significant predictors of histological grade. From this data a CCI has been devised that is practical to use within a clinical setting and which is weighted to take into account the prognostic importance of index cytology and smoking status. Using this type of CCI, a score can be derived for each individual patient, taking into account the important prognostic factors.

# Clinico-colposcopic index – CCI (Shafi–Nazeer index)

| Variable | Score | | |
|---|---|---|---|
| | Zero points | One point | Two points |
| Index cytology | Low grade | – | High grade |
| Smoking status | No | – | Yes |
| Age | ≤30 years | >30 years | – |
| Acetowhitening | Slight | Marked | – |
| Surface area of lesion | ≤1 cm$^2$ | >1 cm$^2$ | – |
| Intercapillary distance | ≤350μ (fine or no mosaic/punctation) | >350μ (coarse mosaic/punctation) | – |
| Focality of lesion | Unifocal or multifocal | Annular | – |
| Surface pattern | Smooth | Irregular | – |

For each individual patient, a maximum score of 10 can be achieved. The higher the score, the more significant the lesion.

| CCI score | Likely histological abnormality |
|---|---|
| 0–2 | Insignificant lesions |
| 3–5 | Mixed histological pattern, often CIN I or II |
| 6–10 | Generally high-grade disease |

## Vaginal extension of CIN

In a minority of patients, there may be extension of the CIN onto the vaginal vault. The colposcopic appearances are similar and the abnormality can be delineated with the use of Lugol's iodine. Atypical epithelium will not take up the iodine stain.

## Endocervical extension of TZ

In some patients, particularly after the menopause, the upper limit of the TZ and any CIN present may extend beyond the colposcopic visual limit. Use of an endocervical speculum may help in visualization of the lower 1 cm of the cervical canal but can be difficult. Excision biopsy, indicated as colposcopic diagnosis, cannot be relied upon if the TZ is not fully visualized.

## Miscellaneous findings

*Condylomata* – These may occur within or without the TZ and indicate infection with HPV.

*Keratosis* – A focal colposcopic pattern in which hyperkeratosis is present and that appears as an elevated white plaque. The white change is present before the application of acetic acid and may preclude adequate visualization of the underlying transformation zone.

*Erosion* – A true erosion represents an area of denuded epithelium. It may have been caused by trauma and may be an indication that the surface epithelium is vulnerable and possibly abnormal.

*Inflammation* – These can produce significant cervical changes particularly hyperemia. Confusion may occur in differentiating inflammatory changes from CIN or invasive disease. If there is doubt, then appropriate biopsies should be undertaken.

*Atrophy* – An epithelial change due to a low estrogen state.

*Polyps* – Enlargement of columnar villi to form polyps. These are usually benign.

*Retention cysts.*

*Deciduosis* – A change identified in pregnancy.

## Unsatisfactory colposcopy

A colposcopic examination is considered unsatisfactory when the SCJ cannot be visualized in its entirety. Examination can also be unsatisfactory if there is trauma, severe inflammation, or atrophy – conditions that may preclude full colposcopic assessment.

| 2011 IFCPC colposcopic terminology of the cervix | | | |
|---|---|---|---|
| **General assessment** | | • Adequate/inadequate for the reason: (i.e. cervix obscured by inflammation, bleeding, scar)<br>• SCJ visibility: completely visible, partially visible, not visible TZ types 1, 2, 3 | |
| **Normal colposcopic findings** | | Original squamous epithelium:<br>• Mature<br>• Atrophic<br><br>Columnar epithelium<br>• Ectopy<br><br>Metaplastic squamous epithelium<br>• Nabothian cysts<br>• Crypt (gland) openings<br><br>Deciduosis in pregnancy | |
| **Abnormal colposcopic findings** | **General principles** | **Location of the lesion**: inside or outside of the TZ, location of the lesion by clock position<br>**Size of the lesion**: number of cervical quadrants the lesion covers, size of the lesion in percentage of the cervix | |
| | **Grade 1 (Minor)** | Thin acetowhite epithelium<br>Irregular, geographic border | Fine mosaic<br>Fine punctation |
| | **Grade 2 (Major)** | Dense acetowhite epithelium<br>Rapid appearance of acetowhitening<br>Cuffed crypt (gland) openings | Coarse mosaic<br>Coarse punctation<br>Sharp border<br>Inner border sign<br>Ridge sign |
| | **Non-specific** | Leukoplakia (keratosis, hyperkeratosis), erosion<br>Lugol's staining (Schiller's test): stained/non-stained | |
| **Suspicious for invasion** | | Atypical vessels<br>**Additional signs**: fragile vessels, irregular surface, exophytic lesion, necrosis, ulceration (necrotic), tumor/gross neoplasm | |
| **Miscellaneous finding** | | Congenital TZ<br>Condyloma<br>Polyp (ectocervical/endocervical)<br>Inflammation | Stenosis<br>Congenital anomaly<br>Post treatment consequence<br>Endometriosis |

| 2011 IFCPC colposcopic terminology of the cervix – addendum | |
|---|---|
| **Excision treatment types** | Excision type 1, 2, 3 |
| **Excision specimen dimensions** | **Length** – the distance from the distal/external margin to the proximal/internal margin<br>**Thickness** – the distance from the stromal margin to the surface of the excised specimen<br>**Circumference** (optional) – the perimeter of the excised specimen |

# Nomenclature

The International Federation for Cervical Pathology and Colposcopy (IFCPC) agreed an international revised nomenclature in 2011. This is reproduced in table format.

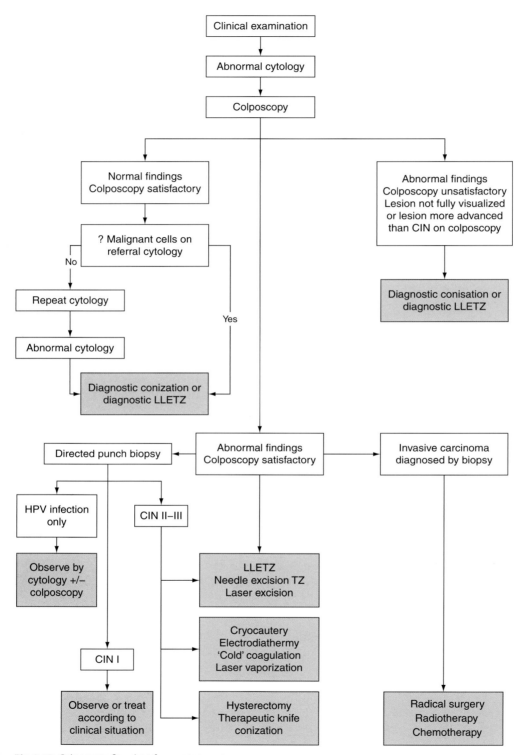

**Fig 4.12** Colposcopy flowchart for management.

## Summary

Colposcopy requires careful evaluation of the TZ. This allows assessment of the distribution of any lesion present including extension to the vaginal vault or endocervix. It aids exclusion of invasive disease and allows characterization between the differing grades of lesion. Colposcopy aids outpatient management of CIN.

## Learning points

- Acetowhite change and assessment of vascular pattern is important for diagnostic colposcopy.
- Many epithelial types display acetowhite change and not just CIN.
- The more intense the acetowhite change and the coarser the mosaic/punctation, the more likely the presence of high-grade CIN.
- Use of a scoring system can aid diagnostic colposcopy.
- Atypical vessels and surface irregularity may indicate an invasive process.

# Chapter 5

# Colposcopic directed biopsies

When a patient is colposcoped and noted to have an abnormality, it often requires confirmation by taking a suitable biopsy. Biopsy is always necessary if the planned intervention is destructive; however, it may not be required if an excisional technique is to be employed. The type of biopsy depends on the clinical situation, degree of abnormality, and need to exclude invasive or glandular disease.

## Punch biopsy

In most clinical situations where invasive or glandular disease is not suspected, punch biopsies will usually suffice. Multiple biopsies from the atypical TZ give greater diagnostic accuracy than a single biopsy. The most severe areas (densely acetowhite, coarse mosaicism, coarse punctation, or with abnormal vessels) of the lesion should be included in the biopsy taking. The biopsies can be sent for histopathological assessment separately labeled as this would affect the clinical management of the patient.

Punch biopsy forceps come in several shapes but all remove a small piece of tissue approximately 3.5 mm diameter. Usually no anesthetic is required; however, the patient's consent is important. The biopsy forceps need to be sharp and able to remove the tissue without distortion. To biopsy a lesion on the margin of the external os, the fixed part of the forceps should be inside the cervical canal and the mobile part outside. If more than one biopsy is required, the posterior lip should be

sampled first in order to avoid impairment of vision because of bleeding. If the lesion lies on the ectocervix, it may be difficult to get a good biopsy sample but with manipulation this is usually possible.

The biopsy should be carefully handled to prevent trauma to, or loss of, the covering epithelium. The crater from the biopsy on the cervix usually requires no treatment. If bleeding persists, it can be sealed by a variety of techniques including vaginal tampon, silver nitrate, Monsel's solution, diathermy or other coagulating process. The patient is advised to expect a vaginal discharge of variable intensity and duration.

## Wedge biopsy

In those women where invasive disease is suspected, a punch biopsy may be inadequate to confidently exclude this possibility. A suitably large biopsy consisting of either a wedge of tissue or cone biopsy needs to be taken. Wedge biopsy is useful when a diagnosis is required without removing too much cervical tissue. A half-moon incision is made with a scalpel over the most suspicious area, including both epithelial surfaces and the SCJ. There is a potential for bleeding with this procedure. Suitable haemostatic techniques should be employed, either by cautery or suturing the edges with an absorbable material. The procedure can be undertaken under local or general anesthesia. A wedge biopsy is not designed to be curative,

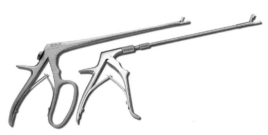

**Fig 5.1** Punch biopsy forceps. Some have rotating mechanism for head manipulation. Handle 'squeeze' mechanism for biopsy.

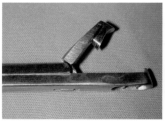

**Fig 5.2** Biopsy forceps detail. These need to be sharp and appropriately sized for suitable biopsies.

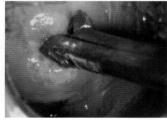

**Fig 5.3** Cervical biopsy being performed.

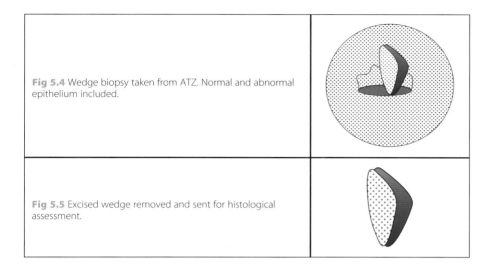

**Fig 5.4** Wedge biopsy taken from ATZ. Normal and abnormal epithelium included.

**Fig 5.5** Excised wedge removed and sent for histological assessment.

whereas a suitably tailored cone biopsy may be. A wedge biopsy is preferred in pregnant women where malignancy is suspected.

## Cone biopsy

A suitably tailored cone biopsy may be used both for diagnostic and therapeutic purposes. Cone biopsy can provide a suitably large biopsy for diagnosis in the following situations:

- Suspected malignancy.
- Glandular abnormality of the endocervical portion.
- Dysplasia is found on cytology and/or endocervical curettage but colposcopy is unsatisfactory.
- Colposcopy evaluation is negative but cytology is persistently positive.
- Upper limit of an apparent lesion is not visible.

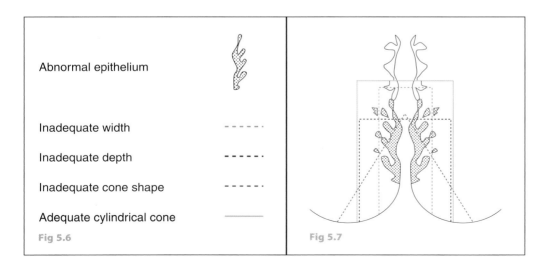

Abnormal epithelium

Inadequate width

Inadequate depth

Inadequate cone shape

Adequate cylindrical cone

Fig 5.6

Fig 5.7

In early invasive disease or for those with completely excised squamous/glandular abnormality, no further treatment may be needed.

Cone biopsies can be undertaken with general or local anesthesia, depending on the choice of technique. A variety of cutting techniques can be deployed including knife (scalpel), diathermy or $CO_2$ laser in cutting mode. The latter two methods can also be used to seal the base of the cone biopsy and provide adequate haemostasis. If a knife is used, the base may be sealed using a pack with Monsel's or the cervical surface sutured. Whichever technique is used, it is important to try and maintain cervical anatomy, as this can be important in the follow-up. Size of the cone biopsy (width and length) affects complication rates. The length of the cone is associated with bleeding complications (primary and secondary) as well cervical stenosis. The width is important for adequate excision of abnormality. The shape will dictate the volume of tissue excised.

## Endocervical curettage

In women where it is difficult to assess the endocervical canal in its entirety but there is suspicion of a lesion residing within the canal based on abnormal glandular cells on the cytology sample or the lesion is extending into the endocervical canal, an endocervical curettage (ECC) can be useful; however, the use and indications of ECC remain controversial.

When indicated, the canal should be curetted using a sharp spoon-shaped or grooved instrument. No anesthesia is required. To obtain an adequate sample the canal should be curetted circumferentially, using short, firm strokes to scrape the epithelium off its base of dense stromal tissue. The criticism of the procedure is with regards to the blind nature of the sample, also the fact that the scrapings are too superficial to give an adequate histological assessment, especially about microinvasion, and may miss disease in the crypts. Moreover, studies have shown sampling with an endocervical brush to be equally informative/efficient, if not more.

## Fixation

Any tissue removed should be immersed in solution of either formalin or Bouins. The choice of fixative is laboratory dependent. Once immersed, the tissue is allowed to fix and solidify over the course of 4–6 hours. After this period of time, it may be removed and trimmed in the laboratory for appropriate histological slide formation, which is stained using Haematoxylin and Eosin prior to assessment by histopathologists. If an excisional biopsy has been taken the dimensions of the specimen and margins should be commented on. The following core data should be available from the histological report:

- Size, state, and nature of the specimen. Mention if there is surgical trauma or coagulation artifact.
- All grades of squamous and/or glandular intraepithelial lesions should be reported and invasive lesions classified and graded.
- Koilocytosis.
- Loop or cone biopsies – has the abnormal squamous epithelium been completely excised (often impossible when loop biopsies received in several pieces).
- Punch biopsy showing CGIN must state that the possibility of invasion cannot be excluded from the biopsy.
- Microinvasive carcinoma cannot be diagnosed on punch or wedge biopsy. A loop or cone containing the entire invasive and intraepithelial lesion is required with disease-free margins to make this diagnosis.
- Microinvasive carcinoma must have the measurements of the invasive lesion reported and indication of Federation Internationale de Gynecologie et d'Obstetrique (FIGO) stage.
- Invasive lesions should have measurements made, margins assessed, and indicate type of tumor, differentiation, and the presence or absence of vascular permeation.

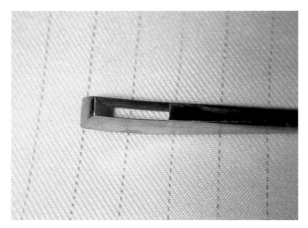

**Fig 5.8** Endocervical curette.

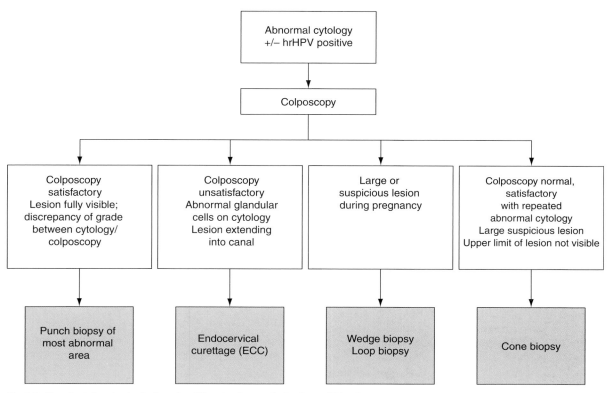

**Fig 5.9** Flowchart showing indications for different colposcopically directed biopsies.

## Learning points

- Cytology, colposcopic findings, and the histology should combine to give a diagnosis in any given individual.
- The biopsy taken should be adequate to make the diagnosis as well as exclude invasive disease if this is suspected.
- Certain biopsy procedures may provide a cure for the disorder.
- Histology reports should have a minimum dataset and agreed proforma can be useful in this respect.
- There is considerable inter- and intra-observer variation in histological assessment, particularly at the lower end of the disease spectrum.

# Invasive cervical disease

The majority of women with cervical cancer will present with symptoms, the most common being vaginal bleeding. Others will present with an abnormal cervical cytology sample of varying degree. The more severe the cytological abnormality, the greater the likelihood of finding invasive disease. Features suggestive of invasion include finding tumor diathesis on the cervical cytology sample.

## Colposcopic appearance

At colposcopy, invasive disease is more likely in large lesions rather than small lesions. Colposcopically, abnormal irregular surface pattern, rolled edges, ulcerative or raised lesions, and the presence of atypical blood vessels are suggestive of an invasive process. These, taken in conjunction with the cervical cytology report and patient's age, are important in forming a colposcopic suspicion of invasive disease.

If invasion is suspected cytologically or colposcopically, the diagnosis must be confirmed by performing a suitably large biopsy. A punch biopsy will not reliably exclude an invasive process and therefore has limited value. A wedge, loop, or cone biopsy will provide enough tissue for diagnosis. With early invasive lesions, a good excisional technique will allow assessment of excision margins and tumor volume, which can inform further treatment plans. A suitably performed loop or cone biopsy may be therapeutic in early invasive disease.

Invasive disease may present as an overt exophytic, fragile mass. In such cases cytology is not useful; an excisional biopsy is performed followed by staging of the disease.

## Staging

The main objectives of staging are to help the clinician plan appropriate management, giving some indication of prognosis. Staging also facilitates exchange of information amongst different treatment centers. Cervical cancer is staged clinically for assessment of tumor

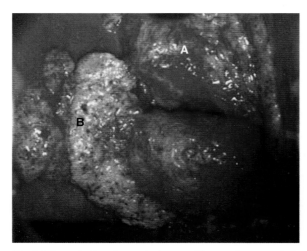

**Fig 6.1** Extensive invasive cervical cancer (A) extending to vaginal fornices (B).

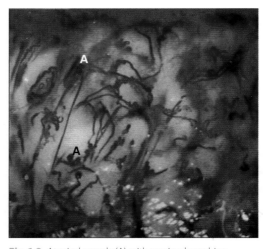

**Fig 6.2** Atypical vessels (A) with varying branching.

In younger women and/or women who wish to retain fertility with a colposcopically visible SCJ, a cylindrical-shaped cervical excision of the TZ and at least 1 cm of the endocervix above the SCJ is recommended. In older women, or those where the SCJ is not visible at colposcopy, the cylindrical excision should include all the visible TZ and 2–2.5 cm of the endocervical canal. If clear margins are obtained, then the CGIN may be managed expectantly. Hysterectomy may need to be considered if clear margins are not attainable or the woman does not wish to retain fertility. It should also be considered in those with ongoing high-grade cytological abnormality after treatment or in those with cervical stenosis, making cytological assessment difficult. Following local treatment, it is recommended that cervical cytology should be performed every six months for five years and then annually for a further five years. Colposcopy is of no value and any residual/recurrent lesion may be more difficult to detect cytologically as compared with squamous lesions. HPV testing as 'test of cure' is not useful as virtually all cases of CGIN are HPV positive. The lesions can be present high in the cervical canal leading to under sampling. Reliance is placed on good quality cervical cytology.

## Issues

As the disease is uncommon, careful assessment of the cervical cytology and colposcopy is warranted. An adequate excisional form of treatment is appropriate and expert histological diagnosis required. Differentiation of preinvasive disease from the invasive lesions is of paramount importance as treatment options are significantly different.

## Learning points

- Adenocarcinoma of the cervix is becoming relatively more important as cervical screening impacts primarily on squamous cancers.
- The natural history of cervical adenocarcinoma and CGIN is less well understood.
- A significant percentage of women will want conservative management of their CGIN in view of their age and fertility considerations.
- Excisional treatments are appropriate for those with suspected or confirmed CGIN.
- Close follow-up after treatment is required with cytology indicating sampling from the TZ including endocervical cells.

# Chapter 8

# Inflammatory and infective conditions of the cervix and anogenital tract

Changes other than preinvasive or invasive disease of the cervix and the anogenital tract can also be seen at colposcopic examination. It is important to understand how colposcopic examination can be beneficial beyond its traditional role of detecting preinvasive lesions. Certain inflammatory and/or infective conditions of the genital region, in particular of the cervix, can mask or make diagnosis of neoplastic changes difficult. On the other hand, colposcopy can help recognize important changes, especially in asymptomatic women, so that appropriate investigations and treatment can be undertaken; however, in asymptomatic woman attending for colposcopy, there is no need to routinely test for chlamydia and other infections. This chapter looks at the inflammatory and infective conditions for which colposcopic examination can be particularly useful.

## Human papilloma virus

Human papilloma virus (HPV) infection is largely transmitted sexually, although evidence of autoinoculation has been documented. All HPV types are epitheliotropic, completing their growth cycle only in differentiating keratinocytes of the skin and the anogenital/oropharyngeal mucosa. There are more than 40 HPV types that are known to infect the human genitalia. HPV can affect the cervix in a subclinical (flat warts) and/or clinical (exophytic) manner causing condylomas. The cervical changes associated with subclinical infections can be similar to those seen in low-grade CIN. These lesions are not visible to the naked eye and become apparent only with the application of acetic acid. Satellite lesions may be present outside the TZ.

In clinical infections, exophytic warts are visible on naked eye inspection. They may mimic a variety of clinical lesions and histological confirmation is

important. The viral type is usually non-oncogenic (often types 6 or 11) and other lesions may be present within the lower genital tract. Lesions may take on some of the characteristics of invasive lesions and excisional biopsy would be recommended in this scenario.

In approximately 70–80% of immunocompetent individuals the infection disappears spontaneously within two years. Treatment of the wart will however, reduce viral load and diminish its ability to transmit the virus to sexual partners. Other indications for treatment are symptomatic cases (itching, dyspareunia) or concomitant epithelial dysplasia proven on biopsy. Various treatment options exist for lesions caused by HPV infection. No single modality is universally successful in eradicating the infection or preventing its recurrence. Most infections respond well after repeated treatments.

## HPV and CIN differential diagnosis

- Precancerous lesions tend to be confined to the TZ, whereas benign HPV lesions may also exist in the native squamous epithelium, sometimes also extending onto the vagina.
- HPV lesions can also present as map-like areas of acetowhitening within the original squamous epithelium.
- HPV lesions can be apparent even prior to acetic acid application.
- CIN lesions in the atypical TZ show some characteristic features – punctations and mosaicism.
- CIN lesions are sharply delineated from the normal epithelium and their distal border is cranial to the SCJ.
- CIN lesions almost always do not stain with iodine.

# Treatment options for HPV infections

| | Surgical | Medical |
|---|---|---|
| **Excision** | **Ablation** | |
| Laser | Laser | Trichloracetic acid (85%TCA in 70% alcohol) |
| LEEP/LLETZ | Electrodiathermy | Podophylline crude extract (25% podophylin in benzoin) |
| Cold-knife | Cryotherapy | Podophyllotoxin 5-Fluorouracil (5FU) Interferons-α and δ Imiquimod |

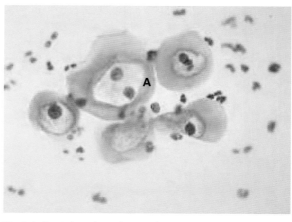

**Fig 8.1** Cervical cytology showing koilocytosis (A) associated with HPV.

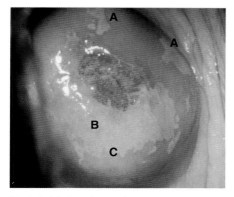

**Fig 8.2** Subclinical HPV infection on cervix – becomes visible following application of acetic acid. Satellite acetowhite lesions (A) outside TZ and minor acetowhite changes (B) with indistinct border (C) consistent with low-grade CIN.

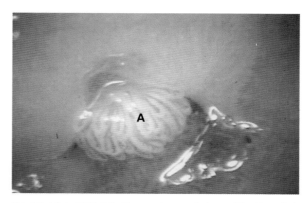

**Fig 8.3** Clinical HPV infection causing cervical wart (A) with typical fronds/micropapillary without acetic acid.

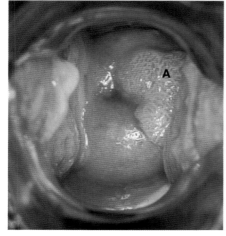

**Fig 8.4** Warty lesion (A) on cervix. These can have variable appearance and are visible in the absence of acetic acid.

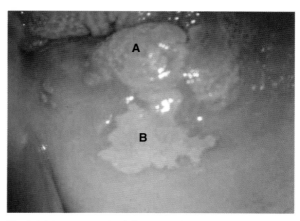

**Fig 8.5** Wart on cervix (A) following application of acetic acid and subclinical HPV or low-grade CIN changes (B).

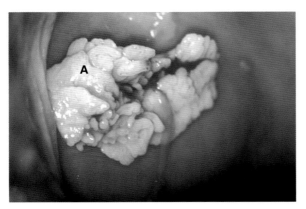

Fig 8.6 Warty lesion (A) encircling cervical canal following the application of acetic acid.

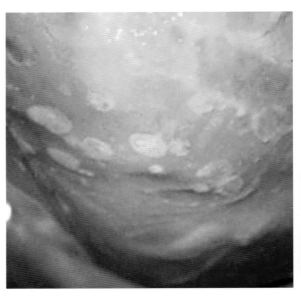

Fig 8.7 Herpetic lesions seen on the cervix in the vesicular phase.

## Herpes simplex virus

Genital herpes is a highly contagious sexually transmitted disease caused by either herpes simplex virus (HSV) type 1 or 2. The former usually infects the oral area often causing 'cold sores'. HSV type 2 is the common infection within the genital area.

Initial infection is characterized by a prodrome of malaise, chills, fever, and enlargement of inguinal lymph nodes. The lesions can occur on any part of the vulva, perineum, or anus. Burning and itching may precede the skin eruption. Typically they appear as one or more blisters/vesicles. The blisters rapidly break, leaving painful, tender ulcerated areas (sores), 1–2 mm in size. The vesicles may coalesce to form large ulcers with irregular borders and pale yellow centre. Dysuria is often present either due to periurethral lesions or herpetic urethritis/cystitis. The lesions reach their maximum size in 7–10 days, thereafter a crust forms with gradual resolution. Complete healing is within 14–21 days.

Further outbreaks can occur but are almost always less severe and shorter than the first episode. Although the infection can stay in the body indefinitely, the number of outbreaks tends to decrease over a period of years.

In 70–90% women with vulvar herpes infection with HSV1 or 2 there is a concomitant herpetic infection of the cervix. This virus causes characteristic lesions on the cervix. The infection can be asymptomatic or can cause ulceration, which may be painful or give vaginal discharge. Biopsy is rarely warranted

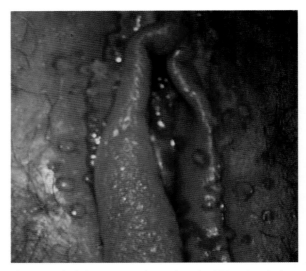

Fig 8.8 Multiple herpetic vesicles on the vulva. This patient had severe discomfort and problems with micturition.

given the history and clinical findings. The infection is self-limiting but its resolution can be hastened with antiviral therapy such as aciclovir, especially if given within first 2–3 days of infection. This is for use on external genitalia only.

## Actinomyces-like organisms

Actinomyces-like organisms (ALOs) detected on cervical cytology do not require any specific intervention in the vast majority of women and are usually associated with intrauterine contraceptive devices (including the levonorgestrel intrauterine system). If the woman is asymptomatic, then an abdominal and pelvic examination is undertaken. She should be advised in relation to a small risk of developing pelvic actinomyces and advised to seek medical help if symptoms develop.

If there are specific symptoms, then the device may need to be removed, after ensuring that sexual intercourse has not occurred in the preceding five days. Relevant symptoms include pelvic pain, deep dyspareunia, persistent intermenstrual bleeding, vaginal discharge, dysuria or significant pelvic tenderness.

Recommended medical treatment comprises a two-week course of antibiotics (e.g. amoxicillin or erythromycin).

## Trichomoniasis

Infection with the protozoa *Trichomonas vaginalis* is highly prevalent in sexually active populations. Although it is considered as a sexually transmitted infection, it is not always the case. It is site-specific for genitourinary tract and can cause vaginitis, cervicitis, urethritis, and pelvic inflammatory disease especially in HIV-infected women. Asymptomatic infection is common both in men and women. Clinically the infection is characterized by profuse, greenish, offensive discharge with erythema, itching, burning, and dyspareunia.

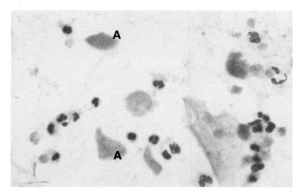

**Fig 8.9** Cervical cytology sample showing infection with TV. Pear-shaped organism (A) with indistinct nuclei.

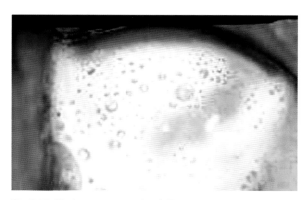

**Fig 8.10** Discharge associated with TV.

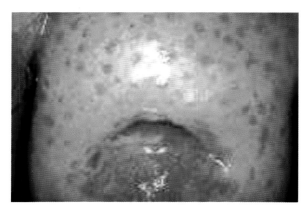

**Fig 8.11** Colposcopic appearance of chronic TV infection showing 'strawberry cervix' pattern.

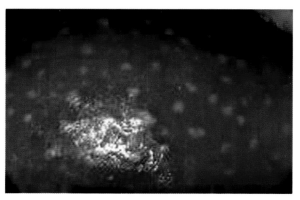

**Fig 8.12** Chronic TV infection on cervix following application of Lugol's iodine to display 'leopard skin' type changes.

41

The colposcopic changes are those of generalized cervico–vaginal inflammation with associated red spots due to cytolytic foci of squamous epithelium with dilated epithelial capillaries surrounded by leucocytes – the changes have been likened to a 'strawberry cervix' or 'colpitis macularis'. After acetic acid the red spots may become prominent. Application of Lugol's iodine gives a characteristic appearance likened to 'leopard skin' with dark background staining of squamous epithelium and failure of staining of the epithelial spots.

Generally, the clinical picture is characteristic. Diagnosis is usually made from wet mount microscopy, directly visualizing the motile *Trichomonas* organisms. The organism may be visualized on the cervical cytology sample with Pap stain or special stain called Diff-Quick. Cultures can be taken from the cervix and vagina.

The treatment consists of nitroimidazole drugs (metronidazole) either in a single dose (2 g) or classical regimen of 250 mg three times daily for seven days. Topical metronidazole is not an effective therapy for Trichomoniasis. The sexual partner should be treated concomitantly.

## Candidiasis

The *Candida albicans* organism is a common vaginal commensal along with the large intestine and oral cavity. Predisposing factors for the development of a clinical infection include: antibiotics, corticosteroids, chemotherapy, oral contraceptives, high carbohydrate diet, diabetes, immunosuppression, and pregnancy. The facilitation into vagina can occur from the rectum, cutaneous foci, or sexual transmission.

Patients with *Candida* infection will often present with vulvar pruritus and thick creamy, cheesy or curd-like, non-offensive vaginal discharge. Examination shows erythema and edema of the vulva and introitus and in severe forms a white pseudo-membrane adherent to the mucosa of vulva, vagina, and cervix. After acetic acid application, fine diffuse whitish patches appear on the vagina and cervix. These patches do not stain with Lugol's iodine.

Clinical picture is pathognomonic for *Candida* infection. Diagnosis can be confirmed on wet mount microscopy with spores and hyphae being apparent in active infection. *Candida* is easily identifiable on cervical cytology especially with gram staining. Culture gives the most accurate diagnosis.

Treatment consists of either imidazole antifungals (clotrimazole) vulvo–vaginal therapy with vaginal pessaries and cream, or triazole antifungals (fluconazole) oral therapy (tablets and cream). Either treatment can be effective both in a single or multiple doses. The sexual partner should also be treated to avoid cross-infection.

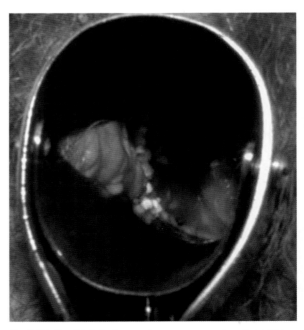

**Fig 8.14** Candida infection can be seen on speculum inspection. Thick, creamy white discharge visible.

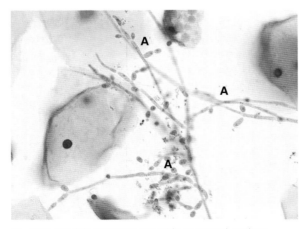

**Fig 8.13** Candida organisms (A) visible on cervical cytology.

# Chlamydia trachomatis

*Chlamydia trachomatis* is the commonest sexually transmitted infection in the UK and perhaps the rest of the world. Up to 1 in 10 women under the age of 25 may be infected in the UK. Women over the age of 25 are also at risk if they have a new sexual partner or have had two or more sexual partners in the previous 12 months.

*Chlamydia trachomatis* is a gram-negative intra-cellular parasite with some bacterial properties. Its different immunotypes are responsible for ocular trachoma (A,B,Ba,C); lymphogranuloma venerium (L1, L2,L3); genitourinary infections, and pelvic inflammatory disease (PID) (B-K).

Most cases of *Chlamydia* infection are either mild or asymptomatic; however, it can lead to an ascending infection causing PID and tubal damage. This in turn can lead to chronic pelvic pain, subfertility and/or tubal-factor infertility, or a high-risk of ectopic pregnancy. Chlamydial infection has also been linked to various obstetric complications such as preterm rupture of membranes and labor. If the baby is exposed to *Chlamydia* during childbirth, then it can develop eye infection or pneumonia.

Diagnostic tests for *Chlamydia* are expensive and technically complicated. Swabs from the cervix or male urethra can be cultured; however, tests based on DNA amplification (polymerase chain reaction, PCR or ligase chain reaction, LCR) are more sensitive and specific and can be performed on cervical and urethral swabs and also first-catch urine from both males and females.

Given the high incidence rates the following categories should be screened:

- All those attending genitourinary clinics and their partners.
- All women seeking or have had a termination of pregnancy and their partners.
- Asymptomatic sexually active women under the age of 25, especially teenagers.
- Asymptomatic women over the age of 25 who have a new sexual partner or have had two or more partners in a year.

Treatment is with doxycycline 100 mg twice daily for seven days. If compliance is a problem, treatment can be with 1 gm azithromycin taken immediately. Partner notification should be routinely performed and every effort made to treat the partner also. Advise 'no sex' until both sexual partners have been treated. Consider screening for other sexually transmitted infections if there is a history of multiple sexual partners.

# Bacterial vaginosis

Bacterial vaginosis (BV) involves an alteration of the vaginal microecological environment and is associated with organisms *Gardnerella vaginalis*, *Mobiluncus* and other anaerobes. These organisms are believed to be essentially sexually transmitted. BV is not caused by poor hygiene – in fact, excessive washing of the vagina may alter the normal balance of bacteria in the vagina, which may make BV more likely to develop. About 1 in 10 women will have BV at some time in their life. Whilst any woman can be affected, it is more common in those with an intrauterine contraceptive device.

In 50% of cases it produces no symptoms. On examination, the vagina is not inflamed, hence the term vaginosis, and there is a thin greyish discharge with fishy odor. When a drop of this discharge is added to a drop of saline on a glass slide with a drop of 10% potassium hydroxide, a characteristic 'fishy amine' odor is released.

Diagnosis can be confirmed by gram stain microscopy showing typical 'clue cells' and absence of *lactobacilli* or by culture. Clue cells are vaginal epithelial cells surrounded by microorganisms.

Treatment is with 250 mg metronidazole three times a day for seven days or a single dose of 2 gm.

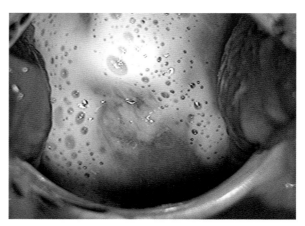

**Fig 8.15** Discharge associated with BV seen on speculum examination.

## Chronic cervicitis

Inflammatory conditions have a varying affect on the appearance of the cervix. The vascular pattern needs careful assessment and the cervix may be tender to touch. Dyspareunia, postcoital bleeding, or vaginal discharge may be the presenting symptom. Possibility of an infective organism should be ruled out by appropriate microbiology. In some of these women, the appearance can suggest an invasive process and recourse to cervical biopsy may be necessary to diagnose the inflammatory process and exclude any invasive component.

In the absence of any specific infection and invasive changes, symptomatic treatment can be given by increasing vaginal acidity and flora (Aci-gel; Gynoflor etc.) or anti-inflammatory agents. Cryocautery or diathermy can be considered in cases of persistent intractable symptoms.

## Nabothian cysts

Whilst these are normal, they can cause concern to the untrained clinician. The cysts occur due to the cervical gland openings becoming covered and mucus collection forming within. Any vessels seen are regular branching (tree-like pattern) and do not justify biopsy. They do not require any treatment and the woman should be reassured.

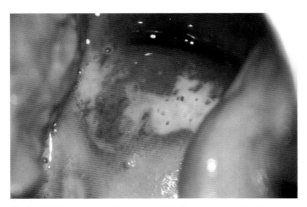

**Fig 8.16** Chronic cervicitis can be difficult to assess with colposcopy and recourse to cervical biopsy may be required to conclusively exclude invasive disease.

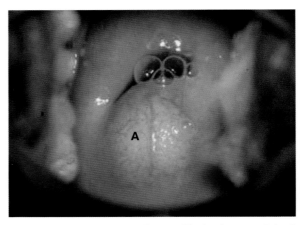

**Fig 8.17** Nabothian cyst (A). Collection of fluid within cervical gland.

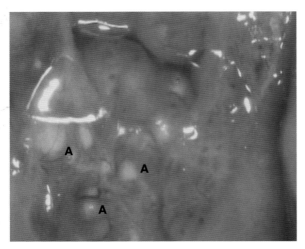

**Fig 8.18** Multiple Nabothian cysts (A), which may appear suspicious for significant pathology.

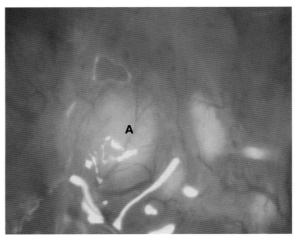

**Fig 8.19** Vessels (A) coursing over the Nabothian cyst seen to be regular with no atypical features.

## Learning points

- Colposcopy is a useful adjunct in those with infections of the lower genital tract.
- Cytology should not be relied upon to diagnose infection.
- Appropriate bacteriological/virological samples should be performed.
- Routine cervical cytology is inappropriate in those presenting with lower genital infections.
- The inflamed-looking cervix or that with warty lesions should be considered as suspicious and invasive disease should be excluded.
- Ablative treatment for warts should only be performed in the context of the woman having a reported normal cervical cytology.
- Young women may present with postcoital bleeding who have an inflammatory condition.

# Management techniques

Treatment is designed with the aim of preventing cervical cancer development by eradicating the preinvasive process with minimal morbidity. An ideal treatment procedure would be:

- Office based
- Cheap
- Quick
- With minimal or no discomfort
- Curative
- With little or no adverse effects (bleeding, discharge, stenosis)
- Followed by good healing
- Allow for adequate cytology follow-up

Two main treatment principles are used, ablation (destruction) or excision (cutting out) of the atypical

TZ. Regardless of treatment modality used, the aim should be to remove the entire TZ.

Ablative techniques include:

- Cryotherapy
- Electrocoagulation diathermy
- Cold coagulation
- $CO_2$ laser ablation

All these rely on heat or cold treatment being applied to the cervix in order to destroy the abnormal skin on the cervix. They can all be performed as office procedures under local anesthesia. Laser treatment is relatively expensive compared to the other modalities.

## Requirements for ablative treatment

- Satisfactory colposcopy – TZ fully visualized.
- Possibility of invasive or microinvasive disease ruled out by adequate biopsy.

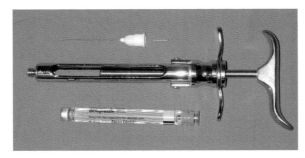

**Fig 9.1** Fine needle (27 gauge size), dental syringe and cartridge of local anesthetic with vasoconstrictor (e.g. citanest containing prilocaine hydrochloride 3% with octapressin).

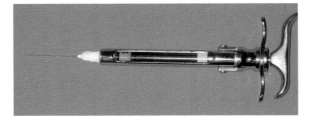

**Fig 9.2** Dental syringe with cartridge loaded and needle attached.

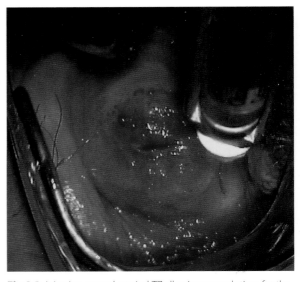

**Fig 9.3** Injection around cervical TZ allowing enough time for the local anesthetic and vasoconstrictor to take effect.

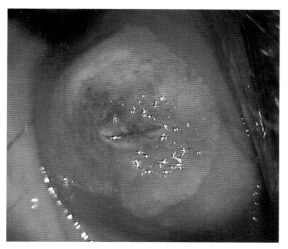

**Fig 9.13** High-grade lesion identified after application of acetic acid involving all four quadrants of the cervix. Local anesthetic injection delivered.

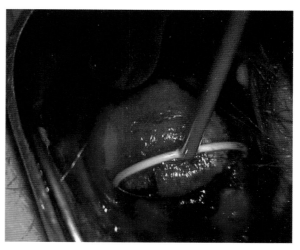

**Fig 9.14** Appropriate loop chosen and excision conducted to a few millimeters outside lesion to ensure complete removal of abnormality.

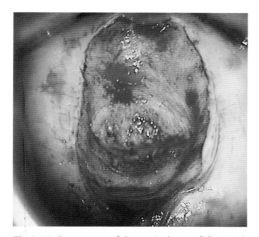

**Fig 9.15** Appearance of the cervical crater following loop excision with some minor bleeding points.

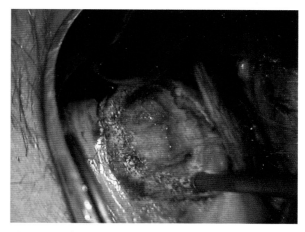

**Fig 9.16** Diathermy ball fulguration or desiccation conducted to achieve haemostasis.

principles of desiccation or fulguration electrosurgery. Desiccation occurs when the electrode or wire is physically touching the tissue and causes more thermal damage. With fulguration the electrode is placed a millimeter or so from the tissue to be treated. This can occur either with the loop when excising or with the ball when gaining haemostasis. Using a blend of cutting and coagulation for the excision, the loop is traversed slowly so that a fulgurative cutting and coagulative effect ensues. If the loop is pushed or a hurried procedure conducted, then desiccation occurs and thermal damage occurs to the excised specimen.

The straight-wire excision of the transformation zone (SWETZ) or NETZ is used when the excision required is asymmetrical or when a large cone biopsy type procedure needs to be performed. It allows the operator to fashion the excision to the individual patient's requirements. The technique is similar to that when $CO_2$, laser, or knife cone excision is performed.

Following excisional treatment, the cervical base is treated to gain haemostasis. A variety of techniques are acceptable. Using a diathermy ball in coagulative mode, the cervix can be treated quickly using either desiccation or fulguration. The rollerball makes this easier to perform as the ball rotates over the surface

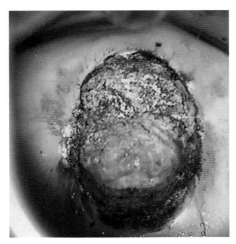

**Fig 9.17** Appearance after cervical crater has been fulgurated. Notice minimal amount of charring.

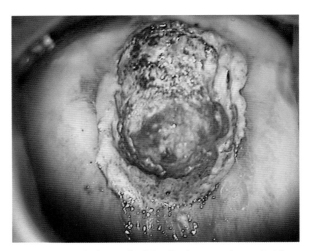

**Fig 9.18** Monsels (ferric subsulphate) solution can be applied for haemostatic purposes. Ideally used in paste format.

and fulgurates the base. With troublesome bleeding, suction, cotton-tips, or jumbo swabs are used to remove/wipe any excess blood and display bleeding points that may require coagulation. Other haemostatic techniques include:

- Oxycel/surgicel or other haemostatic preparations.
- Application of ferric subsulphate (solution or paste). The paste is prepared by aerating the solution over 48 hours, which allows a degree of evaporation to occur. The consistency of the paste can be changed by further additions of ferric subsulphate solution.
- Pack the wound with gauze soaked in ferric subsulphate.
- Silver nitrate.

Following treatment, advice is given to avoid sexual intercourse and insertion of vaginal tampons for four weeks or until the discharge settles. Swimming should be avoided for two weeks. Secondary haemorrhage is usually infective in origin and settles with the use of broad-spectrum antibiotics. Fertility does not appear to be affected following treatment with LLETZ. Obstetric function may be compromised with a propensity to preterm labor and preterm prelabor rupture of membranes, especially in those with deeper excisions (>1 cm depth) or those with repeated excisions. Long-term sequelae are related to the size of the loop, particularly the depth and may be a function of the percentage cervix removed at excision. Stenosis may occur if depth of excision is excessive or repeat loops have been performed.

The histology report should assess the excision margins as this is related to the likelihood of finding residual/recurrent disease. Both the lesion size and excision margins are correlates of follow-up cytology. In those with involved margins, particularly if endocervical, careful follow-up cytology is warranted, including endocervical and ectocervical cytology. In women with involved endocervical or lateral margin who are ≥50 years age, consideration should be given to re-excision where satisfactory cytology and colposcopy cannot be guaranteed. In those with two-margin involvement, there is a much higher risk of residual/recurrent disease and consideration should be given to further excision. Similar consideration to further excision should be given if there is endocervical or ectocervical margin involvement in the presence of stromal-involved margin (i.e. two of the three margins are involved).

## Laser excision

This gives a similar effect as diathermy loop excision; however, it requires greater skill and increased treatment time. High-energy laser beam is used with a small spot size to fashion the excision of the cervical tissue. The treatment may require to be performed under general anesthesia depending on the size of excision required.

## Cold-knife cone biopsy

This technique is still used but mainly reserved for cases where the TZ is not fully visualized, or there is suspected invasive disease or glandular abnormality that requires histopathological ascertainment of the excision margins. The size and shape of the cone biopsy is governed by the colposcopic findings (Chapter 5). The internal os and as much as possible of the endocervical canal are left intact within the confines of disease eradication. This limits haemorrhagic morbidity and fertility will only be slightly compromised, both of these are affected by the length of the cone biopsy.

## Hysterectomy

Some women may need hysterectomy to be contemplated if CIN is present with other gynecological conditions such as fibroids, menorrhagia, or prolapse. Prior to operation, colposcopy will identify the extent of the lesion and avoid incomplete excision, which may result in vaginal intraepithelial neoplasia (VaIN). If the lesion is seen to extend on to the vagina, this may be excised as part of the hysterectomy procedure. A vaginal approach may be ideal to locate the abnormality and excise it in its entirety. If this is not possible, then abdominal approach is utilized taking into consideration the colposcopic findings.

## Learning points

- Ablative and excisional treatments are equally successful in eradicating disease if conducted carefully and with appropriate patient selection.
- Best practice is for a histology report to be available prior to undertaking ablative treatment.
- Depth of treatment should be to a depth of 7 mm to ensure adequate eradication of CIN that may involve gland crypts.
- Cold-knife cone biopsy and hysterectomy retain a place in the management of women with abnormal cytology under certain conditions.
- Audit should be conducted of treatment outcomes to maintain QA.

# Chapter 10

# Follow-up after treatment

Following treatment, all women require regular follow-up for a certain period of time. Women who have undergone treatment for CIN remain at a significantly increased risk of developing cervical cancer (odds ratio (OR) 3–5). In those women that develop abnormal cervical cytology following treatment, the OR for development of invasive disease is 25–30. Close surveillance is required for a number of years and any abnormality during this time warrants a further colposcopic reassessment. If all cytology samples during surveillance remain negative, the normal recall may be resumed.

## Objectives of follow-up

- To ascertain any complications associated with the treatment.
- To detect residual disease.
- To detect any recurrent disease as early as possible.

## Method of follow-up

Ideally, follow-up surveillance should be with cytology and colposcopy. The role of colposcopy in post-treatment patients is still debated by some on the grounds that it can be technically difficult because of scarring, TZ may not be visible in its entirety and the regenerating epithelium is often misjudged as CIN. Cytology has also been reported to give false negative results because the residual disease may be very small or covered by regenerated normal epithelium. Both modalities used in conjunction provide a safety net for early detection of disease.

## Post-treatment complications

Generally, morbidity is very low with all forms of treatment methods. These can be:

- **Early** – excessive bleeding, which may require further corrective management. Most will settle with diathermy or application of Monsel's solution. The Cold coagulator is another useful method of gaining haemostasis. In a small number, suture of the bleeding area may be required. Infection may occur as a secondary event and patients may complain of prolonged vaginal loss, which may be offensive. This generally settles with a course of broad-spectrum antibiotics. No intervention around the time of treatment has been shown to significantly reduce the risk for secondary infection.
- **Late** – Cervical stenosis may occur and is more common after cryotherapy and cold-knife conization. This is particularly the case where sutures have been used as part of the conization procedure. Stenosis is primarily a function of the depth of excision/ablation undertaken, especially if more than 50% of the endocervical canal has been removed. This can be relevant in patients undergoing their second or third treatment. Depending on the degree of stenosis, menstrual problems may occur (amenorrhea, dysmenorrhea) and there will be difficulties in gaining adequate sample for cytology. Fertility problems may also occur. Failure of the cervix to dilate in labor is an unusual complication.

Where cytological sampling is not possible due to cervical stenosis, the options are hysterectomy, cervical dilatation, or withdrawal from further cervical cytology recall with the agreement of the woman. Cervical dilatation should be considered in all cases. In those with a history of high-grade CIN, CGIN, or unexplained high-grade cytology, cervical dilatation or hysterectomy is recommended.

## Residual or persistent disease

Disease that is identified within 12 months of treatment is classified as residual/persistent disease. Abnormalities picked up after this time are usually referred to as recurrent. Most of the persistent/recurrent lesions will be picked up within 24 months of treatment.

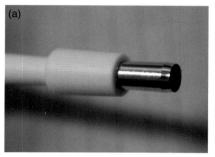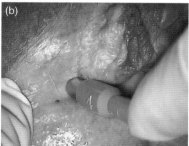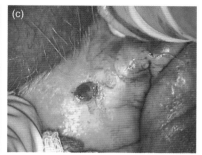

**Fig 12.1** Keyes punch biopsy of vulva being performed. Circular biopsy then can be taken in a variety of sizes, usually 3–6 mm.

Different instruments can be used for vulvar biopsy, which is relatively easy to perform. Biopsy can be taken in an office setting using local anesthetic.

Keyes punch forceps are a suitable method. It removes a round skin area 3–6 mm in diameter. The depth depends on the pressure applied and the thickness of the epithelium. The biopsy site can be left to heal (two weeks). Any bleeding can be stopped by either application of Monsel's solution, silver nitrate, diathermy, or by sutures.

Biopsy is mandatory in the following situations:

- Fast-growing lesions.
- Ulcerations.
- Areas of bleeding.
- Each suspicious area of any color.

## Vulvar carcinoma

Carcinoma of the vulva is uncommon compared to other genital tract malignancies. The exact etiology is unknown but there is evidence suggestive of risk factors that include vulvar warts, which lead to VIN, and inflammatory conditions such as lichen sclerosus and atypical epithelial hyperplasia. The other risk factors include age, immuno-suppression, and smoking. The malignancy risks associated with VIN is 5–10% and 3–5% for lichen sclerosus. The clinical features that may suggest malignant transformation are change or aggravation of symptoms, rapid expansion, or irregular change in the surface contour. Adjacent to vulvar cancers, lichen sclerosus is found in about 60% of cases and VIN (HPV-related) in about 30%.

The most common presenting symptom is pruritus. Other symptoms could be pain, burning, ulceration, or swelling. The lesions are mostly

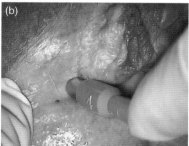

**Fig 12.2** Extensive vulvar carcinoma affecting both labia and invading into the vagina.

multifocal and commonly occur on the labia or clitoris. The clinical appearance may be straightforward comprising of a mass or a suspicious looking ulcer with rolled edges. Small microinvasive lesions in an area of VIN maybe difficult to recognize and in these cases a colposcope can help identify the area, with highest probability of severity, to be biopsied.

If the lesion is small (<2 cm) and unifocal, an excisional biopsy with 1.5 cm of healthy tissue margin can be therapeutic. These women may benefit from sentinel lymph node biopsy rather than formal groin lymphadenectomy. For large or multifocal disease, treatment options are surgical excision, with or without lymphadenectomy of inguinal nodes. Radiotherapy is another option in an adjuvant or neo-adjuvant setting to surgery. Chemoradiotherapy may also be considered for advanced disease.

# Vulvar intraepithelial neoplasia

The exact incidence of different grades of VIN is not known but for VIN 3 it has been estimated to be 2.1/100,000. Substantial increase has been noted over the last few decades especially amongst young women. The risk factors for VIN include multiple sexual partners, recurrent genital infections, immunosuppression, smoking, and HPV. Most cases of VIN 3 are associated with HPV, mainly type 16. Vulvar condylomas are associated with 20–30 % of VIN lesions.

Spontaneous regression of VIN is well documented, especially for the milder forms. Even VIN 3 lesions can regress in the absence of treatment. Regression is most likely in younger women (under 30 years age) with multifocal disease. VIN has malignant potential and the risk of progression is much lower than for CIN (5–10%). These quoted risks are in treated individuals, whereas progression risk may be significantly higher in untreated women. The risk seems to be higher in the postmenopausal age group with unifocal lesions. The true potential of progression, however, is not known. Grading of VIN as 1, 2, and 3 is done along the same lines as for CIN and VaIN.

Unlike CIN, vulvar dysplasia usually presents with symptoms, commonest being pruritus, pain, burning, or dyspareunia. A small percentage will present with a lump/lesion. VIN can affect both hair and non-hair bearing skin. The lesions are usually present on the posterior fourchette, perineum, around clitoris, or lower parts of labia majora and minora. Older women often have a single lesion while young women, under the age of 50, tend to have multifocal or multicentric disease.

The clinical appearance of VIN is variable, presenting in a variety of colors and surface patterns. Typically, they are papular with sharp borders and keratotic rough surfaces. They may sometimes resemble condyloma acuminata. The color varies between white, red, and brown. The diagnosis is always based on histological assessment of an appropriate biopsy. Microinvasive changes may be noted in a significant number of women (16–22%). It is mandatory to do a thorough assessment of the whole lower genital tract including cervical cytology and colposcopy.

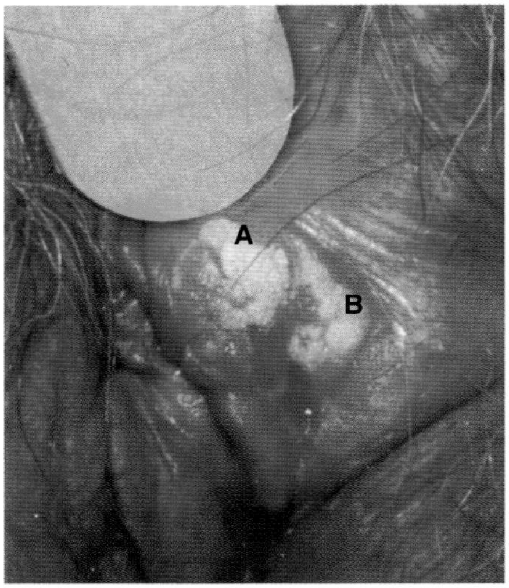

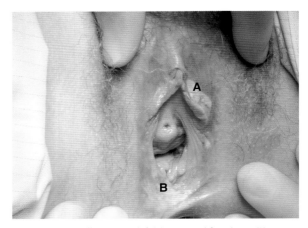

**Fig 12.4** VIN 3 affecting the left labia (A) and fourchette (B).

**Fig 12.3** Discrete area of VIN affecting labia (A and B).

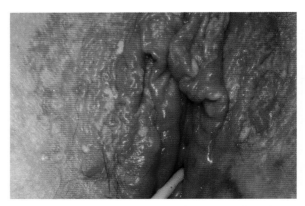

**Fig 12.5** Extensive VIN presenting as erythematous and raised areas.

Treatment is primarily aimed at eradicating symptoms and prevention of potential malignant transformation. A variety of treatment modalities are available. The choice depends on the site, size, focality, and grade of the disease. The age and general condition of the patient are taken into account, as should the preservation, appearance, function of the vulva, and the psychosocial issues.

## Treatment modalities for VIN

- Conservative: surveillance with vulvoscopy and biopsy.
- Medical: 5-FU, imiquimod, α-interferon.
- Laser ablation.
- Surgical:
  - Laser excision;
  - Local excision with knife;
  - Simple vulvectomy; and
  - Skinning vulvectomy and skin grafting.

VIN 1 and 2, because of their apparent low risk of progression, can be managed conservatively. Intervention can be reserved for persistent, recurrent or progressive disease.

Whilst medical treatment may help alleviate symptoms, surgical intervention is important in long-term management. Recurrence rates after laser ablation are high, especially in hair-bearing skin. Local excision is appropriate in the majority of cases and vulvectomy needs be performed in a minority of selected cases. An excision margin of 5 mm of healthy tissue is recommended to reduce risk of recurrence. Post-surgical complications are increased with the radicality of the excision.

$CO_2$ laser still has a place as an adjunct to surgery, especially in young women, to limit surgical damage. It is particularly useful for small areas of peri-urethral and peri-clitoral disease. Laser excision, a more difficult technique, has been described that provides the advantage of laser ablation and offers the possibility of a surgical specimen for histological examination.

## Lichen sclerosus

This is an inflammatory skin disorder whose exact underlying cause is not known. It probably has an autoimmune origin with seemingly genetic predisposition. It is usually seen in the elderly but can occur at young ages. Amongst affected patients, about 15% are

children, mostly girls. There is not much known about the pathogenesis of the disease. The affected tissues retain their maturation potential and the associated atrophic changes are reversible. An association with invasive disease has been reported, with a life-time risk of developing vulvar carcinoma quoted to be 3–5% in women with lichen sclerosus.

Lichen sclerosus mainly affects the vulva but not exclusively. The commonest presenting symptom is pruritus, usually intractable. Other complaints may include vulvodynia, dyspareunia and dysuria. The common sites of affection are the labia minora, inner surfaces of labia majora, clitoris, and the perineum. Lesions may extend posteriorly to the perianal area forming a 'figure-of-eight' pattern. The classical clinical appearance of lichen sclerosus is ivory pallor of the vulva with epidermal atrophy giving a parchment-like wrinkled surface. There is a loss of elasticity and fissuring. As the disease progresses, the architecture of the vulva is distorted, with resorption and fusion of labia minora and loss of clitoral hood. The epithelial surface is waxy, shiny, and speckled. The commonest complications are adhesions and narrowing of the introitus, which may make intercourse impossible.

The clinical features are often straightforward but diagnosis should always be confirmed with an appropriate biopsy. This also helps rule out underlying significant dysplasia or microinvasive disease.

The treatment aims at relief of symptoms and arrest of the atrophic process to prevent complications.

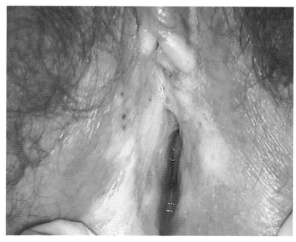

Fig 12.6 Clitoral fusion associated with lichen sclerosus.

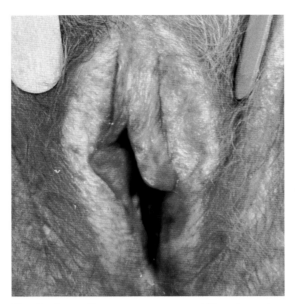

Fig 12.7 Ivory pallor type appearance over labia majora and to a lesser extent the labia minora.

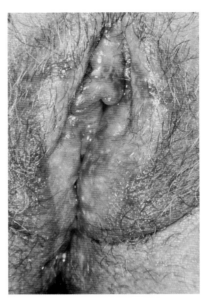

Fig 12.8 Severe changes associated with lichen sclerosus. There is distortion of the vulvar architecture and changes can be seen to extend towards the perineum.

Several treatments have been used but the most effective is the use of potent topical corticosteroids with maintenance therapy at the lowest possible dose. The patient should be advised to use treatment only on the affected areas and could use a mirror to aid application of corticosteroid cream if necessary. Treatment is recommended if there are clinical signs of lichen sclerosus, even if asymptomatic or with mild symptoms, in order to prevent progression. Surgery should be avoided in these cases as it is not more effective than conservative treatments and local recurrences are common. Long-term follow-up is required in view of possible malignant potential.

## Squamocellular hyperplasia

This is a type of vulvar epithelial dystrophy without atypia. Squamous cell hyperplasia is not a distinct entity and is merely a description of the morphologic alteration of vulvar skin. The proposed predisposing factor is chronic pruritus due either to chemical irritation, eczema, or recurrent mycotic infection. Since the causes of squamous hyperplasia are many, they should be properly identified, diagnosed, and treated accordingly. Squamous cell hyperplasia on it own is rarely observed in association with invasive cancer.

When it is associated with VIN or lichen sclerosus, then these women are at higher risk of developing invasive cancer.

These lesions usually present with itching accompanied by red swollen skin. It mostly affects the labia majora, clitoris, and perianal areas. Clinically they appear as thick, dry, keratinised, elevated epithelial patches with diffuse edges. Diagnosis is confirmed on biopsy.

Treatment is symptomatic with withdrawal of the possible irritant, treatment of mycotic infection, topical steroids, and emollients.

## Paget's disease

The vulva is the commonest site affected by extramammary Paget's disease (EMPD), and can either arise as a primary epithelial disorder or a secondary spread from another adenocarcinoma. The invasive potential of Paget's disease has been established but the incidence of progression is unclear.

Typical clinical presentation is erythematous, eczematous eruption with areas of hyperkeratosis. The commonest occurrence is after the age of 60. Common symptoms are pruritus and burning. Paget's disease may exhibit minimally invasive foci but this is not common. It is more notable for its

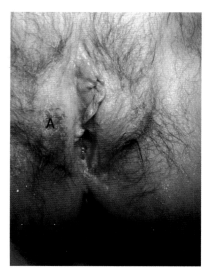

**Fig 12.9** Paget's disease affecting right labia (A).

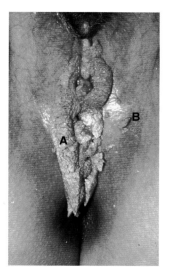

**Fig 12.10** Extensive vulvar warts (A) with some satellite lesions (B).

association (20–40%) with adenocarcinoma of contiguous (anogenital) and non-contiguous (e.g. breast) structures.

Treatment is essentially surgical with wide local excision. Pathological changes tend to extend beyond the clinical borders. Recurrence is common and can be treated with re-excision.

## HPV lesions (vulvar warts/condylomas)

The typical HPV-related lesions on the vulva are warts or condylomas. The incriminating HPV types are 6 and 11.

The mode of transmission is mainly sexual, though autoinoculation has also been reported. The incubation period from the sexual contact to the appearance of lesions can be from one month to three years. Most lesions regress spontaneously but risk factors for persistence or progression are multiple sexual partners, immunosuppression, smoking, and recurrent genital infections.

The quadrivalent HPV vaccine includes protection against HPV 6 and 11 and vaccination has been shown to prevent the majority (90%) of vulvar warts. HPV vaccination against HPV 16 and 18 is effective in the prevention of VIN, which will reduce the risk for vulvar cancer.

## Learning points

- Vulvar conditions usually present as a result of symptoms.
- Vulvar skin is more difficult to assess as there are a wide variety of features associated with vulvar disorders and the vulva is less likely to stain with acetic acid and toluidine blue.
- Neoplastic disease of the lower genital tract is mostly multicentric, therefore evidence of a lesion in one part necessitates thorough assessment of all the other parts.
- Histological confirmation of the disease process is important and can be undertaken in the majority as an outpatient procedure under local anesthetic.
- Treatment of symptoms is necessary as well as the actual disorder.
- Counseling skills are vital in the long-term care of patients with vulvar symptomatology.
- Several vulvar skin disorders can co-exist and some definitely have malignant potential.
- Vaccination is protective against vulvar warts (using the quadrivalent vaccine) and VIN.

# Chapter 13

# Pregnancy and puerperium

The incidence of abnormal cervical cytology is the same as amongst non-pregnant women. The prognosis of dysplasia, irrespective of grade, also remains unchanged. Women should not have routine cervical samples taken during pregnancy if they have had regular screening under a national screening program; however, if a pregnant woman has not availed herself of a screening cervical sample, then this would be an opportunity to perform one. If a previous cervical sample was abnormal and the woman became pregnant before investigation or treatment, then further investigations should not be delayed. The principle aim of colposcopy during pregnancy is to rule out invasive disease and help pursue conservative management until after delivery.

## Normal cervix in pregnancy and puerperium

During the first trimester, the cervix does not appear much different than in non-pregnant state. Under the influence of increased hormones, the cervix is enlarged and softer due to increased vascularity and interstitial edema. This also leads to marked eversion of the endocervical canal. The hypertrophy of the villi and the decidual changes give a polypoid appearance of the columnar epithelium. The TZ is enlarged with marked active metaplasia. There is also thick, tenacious mucus production. All these changes become increasingly prominent as the pregnancy advances. Similar changes are also seen in the vaginal mucus causing edematous hypertrophy of vaginal walls and increased laxity.

## Cytohistological changes

Cervical cytology samples taken during pregnancy and the early puerperium (six weeks post-partum) maybe of suboptimal quality and the risk of false negative cytology is higher. The reason is due to the epithelial changes and the enlarged TZ during pregnancy. In those where there is excessive progestogenic effect, there maybe clumping of cells, making analysis difficult. Decidual change may give rise to the appearance of large cells on the cytology sample which could be confused with dyskaryosis or glandular abnormality.

## CIN in pregnancy

The referral criteria for colposcopy are the same as in the non-pregnant state. Colposcopy is more difficult during pregnancy and certainly more uncomfortable for the woman. They should be advised that colposcopy has no risks to the pregnancy. As the changes in the cervix can be marked, an experienced colposcopist should undertake the examination. The cervix will appear larger and access is more difficult due to positioning and patient discomfort. The area for assessment (TZ) is greater and extensive metaplasia will be apparent. If a cervical cytology sample is performed, there is a greater tendency for contact bleeding and the woman will need reassurance.

Colposcopy becomes progressively difficult as pregnancy advances and is rarely performed in the third trimester, unless there is suspicion of invasive disease. A careful, systematic assessment of all the quadrants of the cervix should be undertaken. The TZ is much enlarged and there is marked metaplastic process. A small area of CIN maybe present in this large area. The acetowhite reactions of CIN (density, mosaicism, and punctation) are more pronounced in pregnancy because of increased vascularity. This can lead to over-diagnosis.

Treatment of CIN is almost never indicated during pregnancy, therefore biopsies should only be undertaken during pregnancy if there is suspicion of malignancy. Punch biopsies are not recommended because the samples are usually unsatisfactory in pregnancy and insufficient to rule out invasive process. The biopsy should be either wedge or cone-shaped and performed in a theatre setting. The intent is diagnostic not

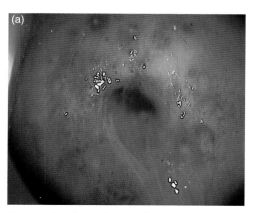

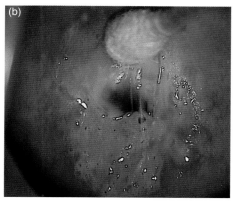

Fig 13.1 Deciduosis changes affecting cervix during pregnancy (before and after application of acetic acid).

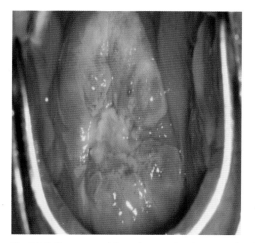

Fig 13.2 Pregnant at 16 weeks gestation. Large cervix with high-grade changes and difficulty in assessing lesion extent and vascularity.

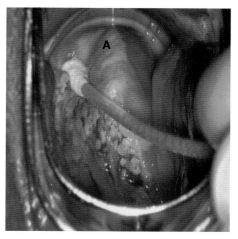

Fig 13.3 Gentle manipulation of cervix to assess lesion extent (A) and rule out any area suspicious for malignancy that may warrant immediate histological confirmation.

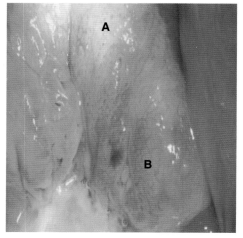

Fig 13.4 Lesion displaying both punctation (A) and mosaic (B) patterns consistent with CIN III.

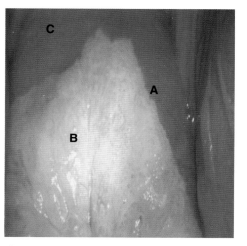

Fig 13.5 Lesion with distinct border (A) between acetowhite changes (B) and native squamous epithelium (C). Coarse punctation present throughout lesion.

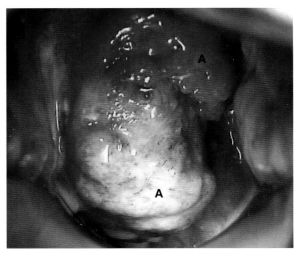

**Fig 13.6** Pregnant woman at 20 weeks gestation with large tumor (A) replacing cervix. Difficult to assess due to tumor size and changes associated with pregnancy.

therapeutic. There is risk of significant haemorrhage and/or miscarriage. If invasive disease is confirmed, the subsequent management depends on the stage of the disease and the gestational age. The decision is made in collaboration with the parents and the obstetrician.

If invasive disease is ruled out, then the management is conservative with cytology and colposcopy, and the decision of treatment deferred till re-evaluation after the delivery, usually 8–12 weeks.

## Puerperium

Women managed conservatively during pregnancy should be re-assessed after delivery within 8–12 weeks. During this time gestational changes on the cervix would have reverted back to normal and any tissue damage resolved. Occasionally, hypo-estrogenic state, especially in those breastfeeding, can make cytological or colposcopic assessment difficult. In such

**Fig 13.7** Flowchart for colposcopy during pregnancy.

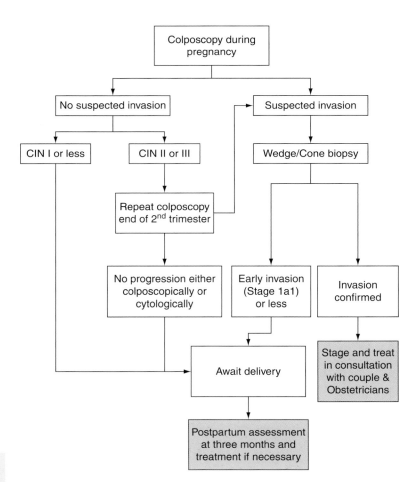

cases, a course of local estrogens (2–6 weeks) may be helpful.

## Learning points

- The principle aim of colposcopy in pregnancy is to rule out invasive disease.
- Pregnancy and the puerperium affects cytology and colposcopic appearances, making assessment more difficult.
- The cervix is larger and colposcopy more uncomfortable during pregnancy.
- The vascular changes can cause overcall of any abnormality present.
- If invasion is suspected, then a suitable biopsy should be performed.
- If changes are consistent with preinvasion, then biopsy and treatment can safely be deferred to the postnatal period.

# Menopause, contraception, immunosuppression, HIV, and smoking

## Menopause

Postmenopausal women remain at risk of cervical cancer. This particularly applies if the woman has not availed herself of the screening program. Those who have had a normal screening history are at very low risk for invasive disease. In the UK, as in many other countries, routine screening for cervical cancer ceases at 64 years. Women therefore continue to have cervical cytology samples for almost 15 years following menopause. However, in the absence of antecedent screening, or if a woman presents with postmenopausal bleeding, a complete cervical assessment along with endometrial evaluation should be undertaken even after age 64.

The estrogen deficiency produces significant changes in the lower genital tract and cervix. There is decreased vasculature and interstitial fluid with flattening of the endocervical epithelium. The TZ appears to recede within the cervical canal. Thinning of the squamous epithelium and reduced mucus production leads to atrophy. The tissue is susceptible to even minor trauma. The epithelium is poorly glycogenated. Taking cervical cytology samples and colposcopic examination are made difficult due to these changes. The inadequate rate for cervical cytology is higher in postmenopausal women as the sampling device has difficulty in reaching the TZ.

## Colposcopic appearance

The indications for colposcopy are the same as in premenopausal women. Colposcopy is made more difficult as the cervix appears atrophic and examination may be more uncomfortable. Examination is more likely to be deemed unsatisfactory as the SCJ recedes and the TZ may not be visualized in its entirety.

The cervix appears small, sometimes flush with the vaginal vault. The squamous epithelium is atrophic and may be traumatized, revealing subepithelial petechiae. Acetic acid may not give significant effect because of lack of vasculature and thinning of the epithelium. On the other hand if the surface is denuded because of physical trauma (speculum, swabbing, cervical cytology sample taking), it may give false appearance of acetowhitening. Application of Lugol's iodine can give a patchy yellow appearance because of lack of glycogen. In older women it may be uniformly yellow because of complete absence of glycogen. TZ is retracted into the endocervical canal because of shrinkage of the cervical stroma.

In those with unsatisfactory colposcopy, the use of local vaginal estrogen (ovules or cream) for a couple of weeks may help to reverse some of the atrophic changes and improve appearance of the TZ, hence allowing a more accurate assessment.

The use of estrogen locally or parenterally in those women with minor cervical cytological abnormalities (borderline or ASC-US), due to atrophic changes, may help improve colposcopic diagnosis in those that are hrHPV positive or those with unsatisfactory colposcopy.

Women with persistent cytological abnormality in the face of unsatisfactory colposcopy (despite estrogen use), or with significant cytological abnormality should have invasive disease ruled out by an excisional

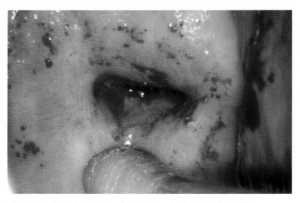

**Fig 14.1** Atrophic cervix showing multiple petechiae. These changes can be reversed with a course of local or systemic estrogen.

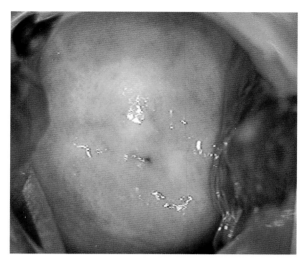

**Fig 14.2** Stenotic cervix in postmenopausal woman.

cone biopsy. In cases of glandular abnormality, the endometrium should also be assessed by ultrasound and endometrial biopsy.

## Contraception

Many women attending for colposcopy will be taking oral contraception. The woman should be advised not to stop taking this, as any abnormality present will not be affected by oral contraception. The changes commonly seen due to hormonal contraception is cervical ectopy, hypertrophy, and a viscid mucus, especially with progestogen-only pills. Sometimes the ectopy can appear quite hyperemic and florid, giving rise to a suspicious-looking cervix, often a cause of referral for colposcopy. In women where the assessment is likely to occur at the time of withdrawal bleeding, women can safely be advised to continue with their oral contraceptives without taking a break.

An intrauterine contraceptive device (IUCD) in situ should not affect the cervical cytology sample or colposcopic examination and treatment can usually be performed without removal of the IUCD. This is especially so for ablative treatments but is also appropriate for excisional treatments such as LLETZ. In a minority, the IUCD will be removed and one should aim to do this in the first half of the menstrual cycle. Alternative methods of contraception will need to be discussed. The IUCD can then be re-inserted 4–6 weeks later at the time of her menstruation. Reinsertion at the time of treatment is

associated with a higher infection rate and is generally avoided.

Barrier methods of contraception (condoms, diaphragm, and cervical cap) have some protective effect against HPV and other sexually transmitted diseases (STD). These should be used in conjunction with a spermicidal that is also virucidal. There is no evidence suggesting benefit with use of barrier contraception in patients with CIN or after its treatment.

## Immunosuppression

This includes women who are on immunosuppressing medication, transplant recipients, and all other forms of immunosuppression. Close cooperation is necessary with other physicians to ensure that the women get the appropriate care they deserve. These women are at increased risk of CIN but this needs to be balanced against morbidity of treatment and the comorbidity of the underlying disease process.

All women aged 25–64 years with renal failure needing renal dialysis must have cervical cytology performed at or shortly after diagnosis. Colposcopy should be performed if resource permits. All women about to undergo renal transplantation should have had cervical cytology performed within a year. Coexisting CIN should be managed according to national guidelines. In women taking immunosuppresants postransplatation, cervical screening should be in accordance with national guidelines for the non-immunosuppressed.

## Human immunodeficiency virus

All women newly diagnosed with HIV should have cervical surveillance performed. Annual cytology should be undertaken with an initial colposcopy if resources permit. Subsequent management should be according to national guidelines. Use of highly active antiretroviral therapy (HAART) reduces HIV viral load and may also reduce HPV viral load. This may reduce the prevalence and incidence of cervical abnormality in such women, but the evidence is inconsistent.

## Smoking

There is evidence to suggest that tobacco can induce carcinogenic effects at sites not directly exposed to cigarette smoke e.g. bladder, kidney, and pancreas. Smoking has also been shown to be associated with increased risk of developing squamous cell cervical cancer. Evidence regarding association with cervical adenocarcinoma is still lacking. There are various proposed mechanisms for this association. Nicotine derivatives and tobacco-specific nitrosamines have been detected in cervical cells. Detectable genotoxic damage in cervical exfoliated cells has also been found. Reductions of local immune mechanisms in the cervix have been shown with decrease in Langerhans cells and other immune markers. Significantly higher rates of regression of CIN have been reported in women who stopped smoking compared to those who continued. In women who undergo treatment, recurrence rates are higher in those that smoke.

Women need to be made aware of these facts and every opportunity should be taken to reinforce the message of prevention. With increasing trends of smoking amongst younger women in some countries,

this could have an important impact on their incidence of cervical cancer.

## Learning points

- Cytology and colposcopy is more difficult in the postmenopausal woman.
- Local or systemic estrogen therapy is useful to obtain good cytology and allow satisfactory colposcopy to be conducted.
- Women can continue with contraception throughout the period of assessment with cervical cytology and colposcopy.
- Women on immunosuppressants or those with HIV are at increased risk for cervical disease.
- Women should be made aware of the risks associated with smoking, not only to their general health but also in relation to cervical disease.

# Further reading

Bornstein, J., Bentley, J., Bosze, P. *et al.* (2011). IFCPC colposcopic nomenclature. http://www.ifcpc.org/documents/nomenclature7–11.pdf

Cancer Research UK (2011). *Incidence-UK, Mortality-UK.* London: Cervical Cancer UK.

Cartier, R. and Cartier, I. (1993). *Practical Colposcopy,* 3rd edn. Paris: Laboratoire Cartier.

Cuzick, J., Arbyn, M., Sankaranarayanan, R. *et al.* (2008). Overview of Human papillomavirus-based and other novel options for cervical cancer screening in developed and developing countries. *Vaccine,* **26**(10), 29–42.

Hinselmann, H. (1925). Verbesserung der Inspektionsmoglichkeit von Vulva, Vagina und Portio. *Munch Med Wochenschr,* 77, 1733.

Jordan, J. A., Singer, A., Jones III, H. W. and Shafi, M. I. (2006). *The Cervix,* 2nd edn. New York, NY: Wiley-Blackwell.

Jordan, J., Arbyn, M., Martin-Hirsch, P. *et al.* (2008). European guidelines for quality assurance in cervical cancer screening: recommendations for clinical management of abnormal cervical cytology. *Cytopathology,* 19, 342–54.

Jordan, J., Martin-Hirsch, P., Arbyn, M. *et al.* (2009). European guidelines for clinical management of abnormal cervical cytology. *Cytopathology,* **20**, 5–16.

Luesley, D. and Leeson, S. (2010). *Colposcopy and Program Management. Guidelines for the NHS Cervical Screening Programme.* Sheffield, UK: NHSCSP Publication 20.

Martin-Hirsch, P. P. L., Parakevaidis, E., Bryant, A., Dickinson, H. O., Keep, S. L. (2010). Surgery for cervical intraepithelial neoplasia, Cochrane Database of Systematic Reviews. Issue 6. Art. No.: CD001318. DOI: 10.1002/14651858.CD001318.pub2.

Petry, K. U. (2011). *Modern Methods for Diagnosis of HPV and CIN in the Prevention of Cervical Cancer.* Bremen, Germany: Uni-med Science.

Richart, R. M. (1990). A modified terminology for cervical intraepithelial neoplasia. *Obstetrics and Gynecology,* **75,** 131–3.

Sasieni, P., Adams, J. and Cuzick, J. (2003). Benefits of cervical screening at different ages: evidence from the UK audit of screening histories. *British Journal of Cancer,* **89,** 88–93.

Shafi, M. I. and Nazeer, S. (2003). Grading System for Abnormal Colposcopic Findings. *In EAGC Course Book on Colposcopy,* eds. P. Bosze and D. Luesley. Hungary: Informa, pp. 33–6.

Shafi, M. I. (2007). European Quality Standards for the Treatment of Cervical Intraepithelial Neoplasia (CIN). European Federation for Colposcopy. http://www.e-f-c.org/pages/recommendationsguidelines/european-quality-standards-for-the-treatment-of-cervical-intraepithelial-neoplasia-cin-2007.php

Shafi, M. I., Earl, H. and Tan, L. T. (2009). *Gynaecological Oncology,* 2nd edn. Cambridge, UK: Cambridge University Press.

Shafi, M. I. and Nazeer, S. (2011). Colposcopy and Cervical Pathology. In *Best Practice & Research: Clinical Obstetrics and Gynaecology,* ed. S. Arulkumaran. Amsterdam, The Netherlands: Elsevier.

Shafi, M. I., Petry, U., Xavier Bosch, F. *et al.* (2011). European consensus statement on 'HPV vaccination and colposcopy'. *Journal of Lower Genital Tract Disease,* 15(4), 309–15.

Solomon, D., Davey, D., Kurman, R. *et al.* (2002). The 2001 Bethesda System: terminology for reporting results of cervical cytology. *Journal of American Medical Association,* **287,** 2114–19.

WHO position paper, (2009). Human papillomavirus vaccines. *Biologicals,* **37**(5), 338–44.

Wright, T. C., Massad, L. S., Dunton, C. J., Spitzer, M., Wilkinson, E. J. and Solomon, D. (2006). ASCCP sponsored consensus conference. 2006 consensus guidelines for the management of women with abnormal cervical screening tests. *Journal Lower Genital Tract Disease,* **11**(4), 201–22.

# Index